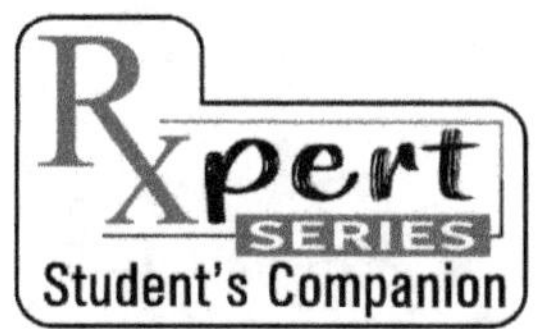

Human Anatomy and Physiology
- A Practical Manual

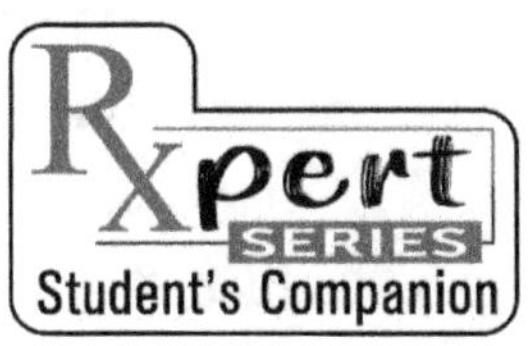

Human Anatomy and Physiology
- A Practical Manual

Havagiray R. Chitme
Professor of Pharmacology & Head, IPR Cell
DIT University, Dehradun

Ajay Kumar Gupta
Associate Professor of Pharmacology
C. S. J. M. University, Kanpur

Anuj Nautiyal
Associate Professor of Pharmacy Practice
S. G. R. R. University, Dehradun

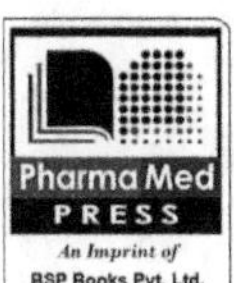

PharmaMed Press
An imprint of BSP Books Pvt. Ltd.
4-4-309/316, Giriraj Lane,
Sultan Bazar, Hyderabad - 500 095.

Human Anatomy and Physiology - A Practical Manual

by Havagiray R. Chitme, Ajay Kumar Gupta, Anuj Nautiyal

Published by

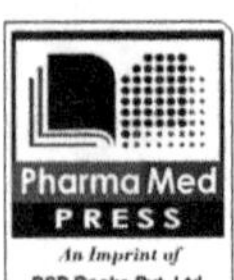

PharmaMed Press

An imprint of BSP Books Pvt. Ltd.

4-4-309/316, Giriraj Lane, Sultan Bazar, Hyderabad - 500 095.
Phone: 040-23445688; Fax: 91+40-23445611
E-mail: info@pharmamedpress.net
www.bspbooks.net/www.pharmamedpress.net

ISBN: 978-93-95039-41-3 (Paperback)

PREFACE

Human Anatomy and Physiology - A Practical Manual is written with one of the most easily understandable language for Diploma in Pharmacy students as per the ER-20 syllabus of Pharmacy Council of India. Each experiment is structured with objective, requirements, principle, procedure, observation and results. There are totally 36 experiments covering almost all body systems. The last chapter on Viva Voce help the students to prepare themselves for synopsis and viva voce of external practical examination. This manual also help in preparing the students for proposed D. Pharm exit examination.

This manual also contains pictures/images to facilitate learning and ease to understand the concepts. The normal values placed for some of the experiments will help the students to understand the physiological abnormalities. The step-wise description of the procedure will help the students to follow them systematically and get the results. The theory involved in each experiment is given as principle to synchronise the theoretical learning and practical experience to enhance the practice of learning by doing.

This manual is the result and encouragement received from our own teaching and research experience in the field of pharmacy and other health care profession. We are hopeful and confident that it will be reviewed and edited on regular basis to improvise learning experience of students. We are also grateful to our publishers and their editorial board for their cooperation, encouragement and suggestions.

We hope this manual will be found very useful by the students and teachers.

March, 2023 *-Authors*

Contents

Experiment No: 1

Study of Compound Microscope

Objective:	To study the various parts and draw the compound microscope
Requirement:	Compound microscope

Principle

The compound microscope has a combination of lenses that enhances both magnifying power as well as the resolving power. The specimen or object, to be examined is usually mounted on a transparent glass slide and positioned on the specimen stage between the condenser lens and objective lens.

A beam of visible light from the base is focused by a condenser lens onto the specimen. The objective lens picks up the light transmitted by the specimen and create a magnified image of the specimen called primary image inside the body tube. This image is again magnified by the ocular lens or eye piece.

The compound microscope is called so because, in contrast to a single magnifying convex lens, it has two such lenses-the objective and the eyepiece. It magnifies the image of an object that is not visible to the naked eye to an extent where it can be seen clearly.

Procedure

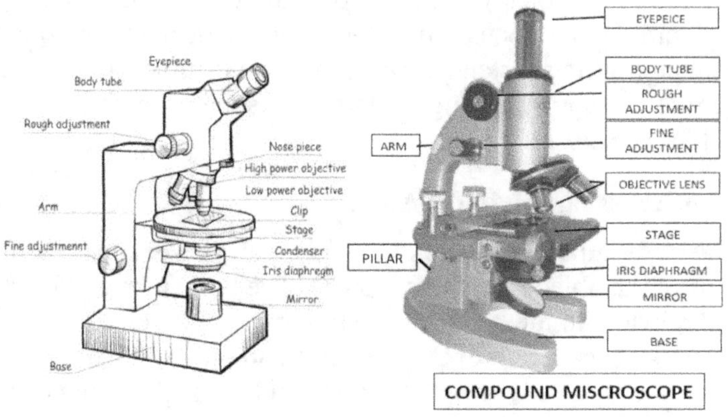

Study the following parts of compound microscope as follows:

A. The support system

B. The focusing system

C. The optical system (magnification system)

D. The illumination system

A. The Support system

1. **Base:** It is a heavy-metallic, U-or horseshoe-shaped base or foot, which supports the microscope on the working table to provide maximum stability.

2. **Pillars**: Two upright pillars project up from the base and are attached to the C-shaped handle. The hinge joint allows the microscope to be tilted at a suitable angle for comfortable viewing.

3. **Handle (arm or limb):** The curved handle, which projects up from the hinge joint supports the focusing and magnifying system.

4. **Body tube:** fitted at the upper end of the handle, either vertically or at an angle, the body tube is the part through which light passes to the eyepiece. It can be raised or lowered by the focusing system.

5. **The stage:** It is a rectangular/square flat platform with an aperture in its center, and fitted to the arm below the objective lenses. The slide is placed on it and centered over the aperture for viewing. The light emerging from the condenser passes through the slide and objective into the body tube.

B. The Focusing system

It consists of two coarse and two fine adjustment screw-heads: It is employed for raising or lowering the optical system with reference to the slide till it comes to the focus. Thus, the adjustments place an objective lens at its optimal working distance. The coarse adjustment moves the optical system up down rapidly through a large distance. The fine adjustment is employed for precise focusing.

C. The Optical (Magnifying) system

1. **The body tube:** It is a hollow tubular part present between the upper ends of the objectives and eyepiece. The body tube can be moved up and down with the help of adjustment screws. The distance between the upper focal point of the eyepiece and the lower focal point of the objective is called the optical tube length, which is about 25cm.

2. **Eyepiece:** It fits into the top of the body tube and through it an image is seen. Most microscopes are provided with replaceable 5x, 8x, and 10x eyepieces, though 6x and 15x are also available. Each eyepiece has two lenses- one mounted at the top, **the eye lens** and the other, the **field lens,** is fitted at the bottom. The field lens collects the divergent rays of the primary image and passes these to the eye lens, which further magnifies the image.

3. **The nosepiece:** It is a circular metallic structure fitted at the lower end of the body tube and has fixed and revolving nosepiece. The revolving nosepiece carries interchangeable objective lenses. Its correct position being indicated by a click sound.

4. **Objective lenses:** The magnifying power of each lens and its numerical aperture (NA) provided rather than its focal length are written on each lens.

   a) *Low-power objective (10x: NA= 0.25)*: This lens magnifies the image 10 times. It is used for initial focusing and viewing a large area of the specimen slide.

   b) *High-power objective (45x: NA=0.65)*: This lens magnifies the image 45 times. Because of higher magnification, it is used for more detailed study of the material.

   c) *Oil-immersion objective (100x: NA=1.30)*: This lens magnifies the image 100 times. Since the lens almost touches the slide it has to be immersed in a special medium (cedar wood oil), a drop of which is first placed on the slide. The oil is used to increase the NA and thus the resolving power of the objective. As this lens gives a total magnification of 1000 times, it is employed for detailed study of blood cells and tissues.

D. The illumination system

1. **Source of light**: The source of light may be the diffuse, natural day light (sunlight) reflected and scattered by the atmosphere and its dust particles and reflected from the buildings. On bright, sunny days, the day light is the ideal for routine student work.

   If day light is not available, or is not sufficient, an artificial source of light a fluorescent tube fitted on the working table can provide enough light.

2. **The mirror**: A double sided mirror, in fact two mirrors, one flat or plane and the other concave, fitted back to back in a metal frame is located below the condenser. It can be rotated in any direction. The

plane mirror is used with a distant natural source of light. The concave mirror is used when the light source is near the microscope.

3. **The condenser**: It is a system of lenses fitted in a short cylinder that is mounted below the stage. It can be raised or lowered by a rack and pinion, and focusing the light rays into a solid core of light on to the material under study. It also helps in resolving the image.

a) The lens system: It is composed of two lenses. Since the condenser is a lens system, it has a fixed NA, which should be equal or less than that of the objective being used. With axes of the two being the same, all the light passing through the condenser is collected by the objective, thus allowing maximum clarity.

b) The iris diaphragm: It is fitted within the condenser to adjust the size of the aperture of the diaphragm and regulate the intensity of the light falling on the material under study.

Observation: Observe and draw a neat labelled diagram of compound microscope and measure the length of body tube, number of objectives, magnification of eyepiece, and type of stage.

Precautions

1. Always keep compound microscope in an upright position.
2. Avoid touching lenses with your hands.
3. Keep the microscope covered or in box, when not in use.

Result: Compound microscope studied in detail and its diagram has been drawn. A table of observation is made and values are recorded.

Experiment No: 2

General Techniques of Blood Collection

Objective:	To study the general techniques for the collection of blood
Requirement:	Syringe, needle, glass slides, cotton

PRINCIPLE

BLOOD SAMPLING

There are several methods of collection of blood. Following are the two most common methods:

Venipuncture

Advantages:

  (i)   Recommended for collecting large quantity of venous blood
  (ii) The composition of blood is not significantly different from that of the capillary blood
  (iii) Blood is obtained by a single puncture and repeated investigations can be carried out

Disadvantages:

The procedure requires a technical person with

  (i)   Skill and confidence
  (ii) May also require assistance
  (iii) Individuals to be cooperative
  (iv) Complete aseptic precautions and
  (v)   Anticoagulant containers (vacutainer)

Prick Method: The method is used when only couple of drops of blood is sufficient/required.

Site for Pricking: A vascular site under good physical control is chosen. Pad of the thumb or great toe or the heel in infants and the ball of a finger or the lobe of either ear in adults are the common sites. The skin of the part selected should be healthy and not be edematous, congested, bloodless, or cold. The pricking should not be undertaken if it is not possible to observe the aseptic precautions.

PROCEDURE

Venipuncture:

1. Let the subject lie down on the bed or sit on a chair to relax.
2. Reassure the patient/ individual and put him/her to ease.
3. Examine the cubital fossa of his left arm for a "suitable vein".
4. Obstruct the venous return either with the armlet of a blood pressure apparatus raising the pressure to 40 mm Hg level or with a strap of broad elastic or by compression of the arm above the vein.
5. Rest the fully extended arm comfortably on padding.
6. Clean the skin over the selected vein with spirit and allow it to dry.
7. Fix the selected vein by traction on the skin over it with the thumb of your left hand
8. Hold the syringe along the vein and the level of the needle.
9. Place your first finger nearest to the butt of the needle and the body of the syringe in the palm of your hand.
10. Locate a spot on the vein about half a cm below its maximal turgor pressure.
11. Puncture at the spot by pushing in the needle firmly and steadily forming an angle of 30° to 50° with the lower arm.
12. When you have punctured the skin, the resistance encountered is suddenly reduced.
13. Put a slight drag on the piston with your little or ring finger to induce a little negative pressure in the syringe.
14. Push the needle along the line of the vein and if necessary at a changed angle to puncture the vein.
15. When the vein is punctured blood enters the syringe and the resistance encountered for pulling the piston is suddenly reduced.
16. Fix the syringe with left hand and slowly withdraw piston with the right hand as the blood enters the syringe.

17. When sufficient amount of blood is withdrawn hold the syringe in the palm the little and ring fingers supporting the piston and the index finger on the butt of the needle.

18. Place a piece of sterile cotton wool soaked in spirit on the punctured site with the left hand and press lightly.

19. Withdraw the needle with the syringe and press the swab firmly on the punctured site.

20. Instruct the subject to hold it pressed.

21. Hold the syringe vertical with the piston supported.

22. Hold the collection tube with the left hand and slowly transfer the blood in it.

23. Discard the syringe and needle safely as per the guidelines.

24. Hold the collection tube in the palms of your hands and rotate it forwards & backward till the anticoagulant thoroughly mixes.

25. Label the container and keep aside for testing.

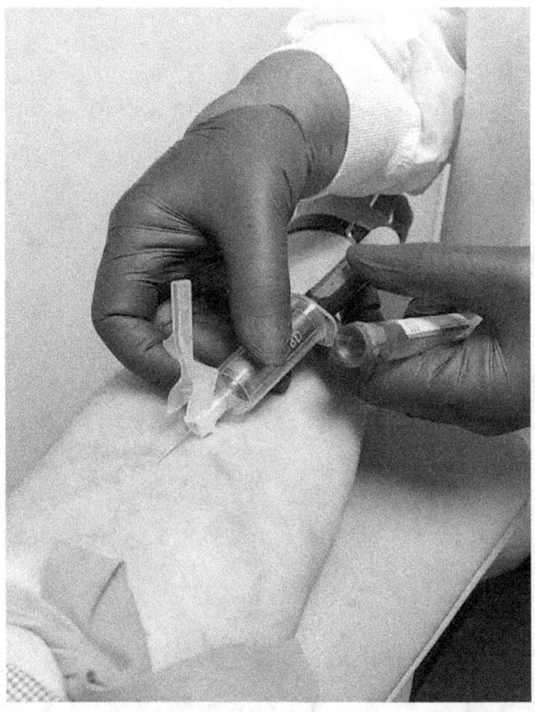

Obtaining Sample by the Prick Method

1. Clean and massage the finger with a dry clean sterile gauze swab soaked in methylated spirit.
2. Dip the left-hand ring finger in warm water at 40° C for 3 to 5 minutes or rub the finger to facilitate the flow of blood.
3. Allow the finger to get dry.
4. Hold the finger to be pricked in your left hand.
5. Press the ball of the finger to raise the skin into a small ridge in the longitudinal axis.
6. Hold the disposable sterile lancet with the right-hand fingers.
7. Hold the finger so that the puncture faces you.
8. Mop the oozed plasma and first part of blood.
9. Wipe the lancet, clean and then dispose it.
10. Allow a drop of about 3 mm diameter of blood formed on the punctured site.
11. Collect it as desired.
12. When blood is collected successfully, apply a sterile gauze swab soaked in spirit and keep the site pressed for 1 minute or till the bleeding ceases.

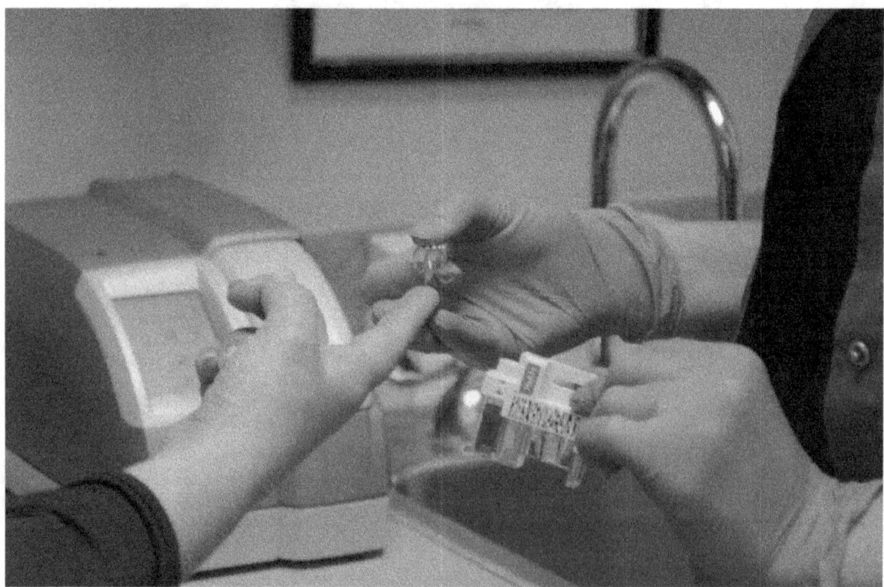

Precautions

1. Wash your hands, clean with plenty of soap and water and dry them with a sterilized cloth piece or tissue paper.
2. Confirm that the packet of the irradiated sterilized syringe and the needle are sealed.
3. Do not touch the cutting portion of the sterile lancet or syringe needle or the site of the finger to be pricked or punctured.
4. Do not force blood collected in syringe into container through the needle as it causes hemolysis.
5. The back and forth movement of container for mixing with anticoagulant should not be too vigorous as it causes hemolysis.
6. Label the container with care to avoid error in labeling patient/ individual ID.

Observation: The students will observe both methods of blood collection and write their observation with respect to ease of collection, advantages, disadvantages, and challenges.

Result: Blood collection techniques have been performed and learned.

Experiment No: 3

Microscopic Examination of Epithelial Tissue

Objective:	To study and draw the microscopic structure of epithelial tissue
Requirements:	Charts /models/slides of epithelial tissues, compound microscope

Theory

Tissue is a group of similar cells that usually have a common origin and functions together to carry out specialized activities. Epithelial tissue covers the body surfaces and lines hollow organs, body cavities, ducts and forms glands. Epithelial tissues are classified according to following two characteristics:

1. the arrangement of cells into layers and
2. the shapes of the cells

By studying the microscopy of epithelial tissues, the structure of different types of epithelial tissues could be understood.

Procedure

Collect the chart or tissue slide and observe the slides of different epithelial tissues under compound microscope and observe their structure, arrangement with respect to their function as follows:

A) **Arrangement of cells in layers**: The cells are arranged in one or more layers depending on the functions the epithelium performs:

   a. **Simple epithelium** is a single layer of cells that functions in diffusion, osmosis, filtration, secretion, or absorption. Secretion is the production and release of substances such as mucus, sweat, or enzymes. Absorption is the intake of fluids or other substances such as digested food from the intestinal tract.

   b. **Pseudostratified epithelium** (pseudo = false) appears to have multiple layers of cells because the cell nuclei lie at different levels and not all cells reach the apical surface. Cells that do extend to the apical surface may contain cilia; others (goblet cells) secrete mucus. Pseudostratified epithelium is actually a simple epithelium because all its cells rest on the basement membrane.

c. Stratified epithelium (stratum = layer) consists of two or more layers of cells that protect underlying tissues in locations where there is considerable wear and tear.

B) Cell shapes: The cells vary in shape depending on their function.

(a) **Squamous cells** (flat) are arranged like floor tiles and are thin, which allows for the rapid passage of substances.

(b) **Cuboidal cells** are as tall as they are wide and are shaped like cubes or hexagons. They may have microvilli at their apical surface and function in either secretion or absorption.

(c) **Columnar cells** are much taller than they are wide, like columns, and protect underlying tissues. Their apical surfaces may have cilia or microvilli, and they often are specialized for secretion and absorption.

(d) **Transitional cells** change shape, from flat to cuboidal and back, as organs such as the urinary bladder stretch (distend) to a larger size and then collapse to a smaller size.

C) Combining the two characteristics (arrangements of layers and cell shapes)

1. Simple epithelium

   1.1 Simple squamous epithelium

   1.2 Simple cuboidal epithelium

   1.3 Simple non-ciliated columnar epithelium

   1.4 Simple ciliated columnar epithelium

   1.5 Pseudostratified columnar epithelium (non-ciliated and ciliated)

2. Stratified epithelium

   2.1 Stratified squamous epithelium (keratinized and nonkeratinized)

   2.2 Stratified cuboidal epithelium

   2.3 Stratified columnar epithelium

   2.4 Transitional epithelium

   1.1 Simple Squamous epithelium:

      Description: Single layer of flat cells; centrally located nucleus.

Location: Lines heart, blood vessels, lymphatic vessels, air sacs of lungs, glomerular (Bowman's) capsule of kidneys, and inner surface of the tympanic membrane (eardrum); forms epithelial layer of serous membranes, such as the peritoneum, pericardium, and pleura.

Function: Filtration, diffusion, osmosis, and secretion in serous membranes

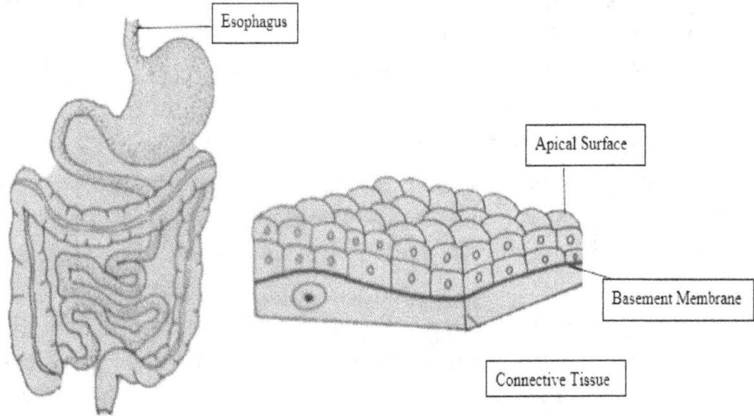

1.2   Simple Cuboidal epithelium:

Description: Single layer of cube-shaped cells; centrally located nucleus.

Location: Covers surface of ovary, lines anterior surface of capsule of the lens of the eye, forms the pigmented epithelium at the posterior surface of the eye, lines kidney tubules and smaller ducts of many glands, and makes up the secreting portion of some glands such as the thyroid gland and the ducts of some glands such as the pancreas.

Function: Secretion and absorption

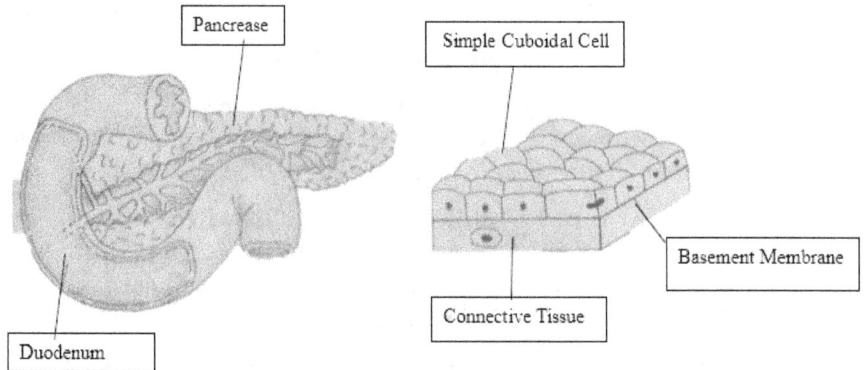

1.3   Simple non-ciliated columnar epithelium: -

Description: Single layer of non-ciliated column-like cells with nuclei near base of cells; contains goblet cells and cells with microvilli in some locations.

Location: Lines the gastrointestinal tract (from the stomach to the anus), ducts of many glands, and gallbladder.

Function: Secretion and absorption

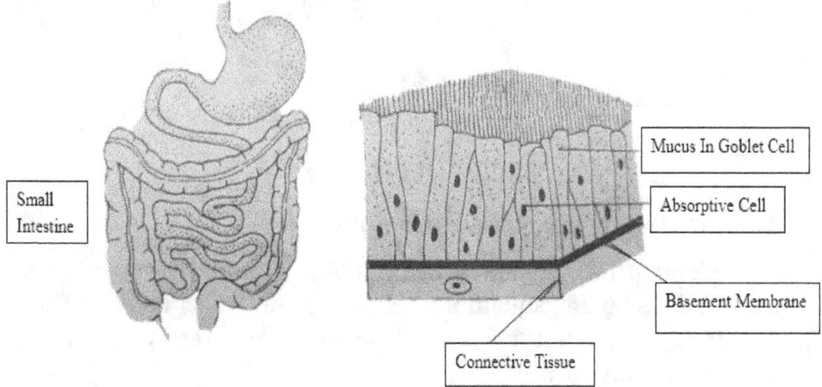

1.4   Simple Ciliated columnar epithelium: -

Description: Single layer of ciliated column-like cells with nuclei near base; contains goblet cells in some locations.

Location: Lines some bronchioles (small tubes) of respiratory tract, uterine (fallopian) tubes, uterus, efferent ducts of the testes, some paranasal sinuses, central canal of spinal cord, and ventricles of the brain.

Function: Moves mucus and other substances by ciliary action

1.5   Pseudostratified columnar epithelium

Description: Not a true stratified tissue; nuclei of cells are at different levels; all cells are attached to basement membrane, but not all reach the apical surface.

Location: Pseudostratified ciliated columnar epithelium lines the airways of most of upper respiratory tract; pseudostratified nonciliated columnar epithelium lines larger ducts of many glands, epididymis, and part of male urethra.

Function: Secretion and movement of mucus by ciliary action.

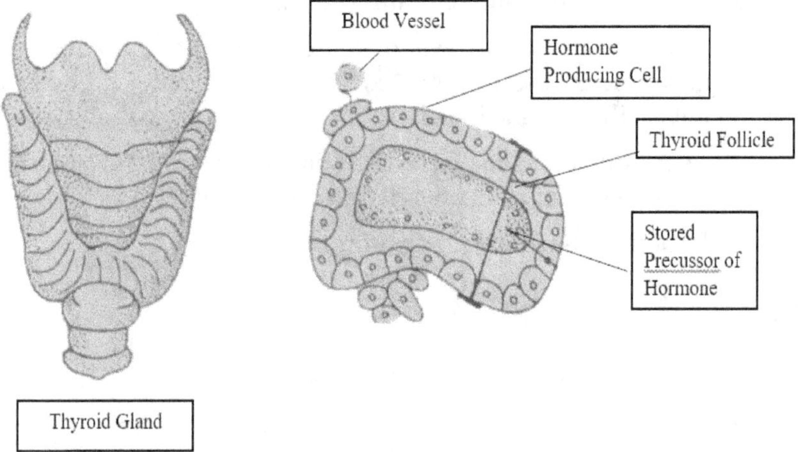

2.1   Stratified squamous epithelium

Description: Several layers of cells; cuboidal to columnar shape in deep layers; squamous cells form the apical layer and several layers deep to it; cells from the basal layer replace surface cells as they are lost.

Location: Keratinized variety forms superficial layer of skin; nonkeratinized variety lines wet surfaces, such as lining of the mouth, esophagus, part of larynx, part of pharynx, and vagina, and covers the tongue.

Function: Protection

2.2 Stratified cuboidal epithelium

Description: Two or more layers of cells in which the cells in the apical layer are cube-shaped.

Location: Ducts of adult sweat glands and esophageal glands and part of male urethra.

Function: Protection and limited secretion and absorption.

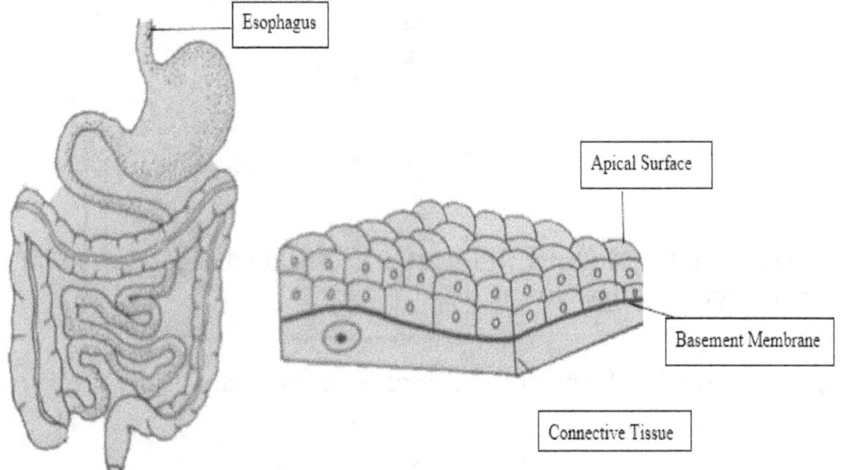

2.3 Stratified columnar epithelium

Description: Several layers of irregularly shaped cells; only the apical layer has columnar cells.

Location: Lines part of urethra, large excretory ducts of some glands, such as esophageal glands, small areas in anal mucous membrane, and part of the conjunctiva of the eye.

Function: Protection and secretion

2.4 Transitional epithelium:

Description: Appearance is variable (transitional); shape of cells in apical layer ranges from squamous (when stretched) to cuboidal (when relaxed).

Location: Lines urinary bladder and portions of ureters and urethra.

Function: Permits distension.

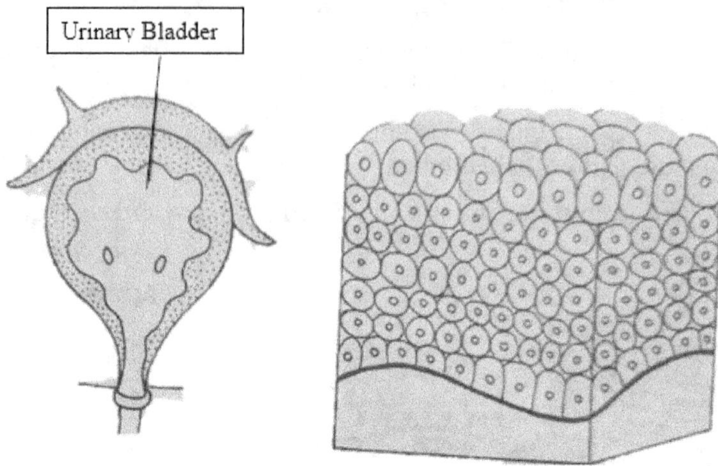

Observation: The students will draw a neat and labelled diagram of the different types of connective tissue.

Result: Study of differential characteristics of epithelial tissue was carried out.

Experiment No: 4

Microscopic Examination of Cardiac Muscle

Objective:	To study the microscopic features of cardiac muscle using compound microscope
Equipment/ Glassware Required:	Charts/models/slides of cardiac muscle/compound microscope

Principle

Cardiac muscles present only in heart are similar to skeletal muscle but they are beyond our control i.e. autonomous in their function. Cardiac muscle surrounds the chambers of the heart and is used to pump blood through the body. Unlike skeletal muscle, cardiac muscle fibers are arranged in a branching pattern instead of a linear pattern. Both skeletal muscle and cardiac muscle need to contract quickly and often, which is why the striations can be seen. Their electrical, mechanical and autonomous nature makes them different from any other muscles and tissues. Cardiac muscles continuously function throughout life without getting tired.

Procedure

Collect the chart or tissue slide and observe the slides of cardiac muscle under compound microscope and observe their structure, arrangement with respect to their function as follows:

1. Both longitudinal and transverse striations
2. The location of nucleus and its pattern
3. Characteristic presence of intercalated disc
4. Place of branching of cardiac muscles
5. Draw the observation and label it

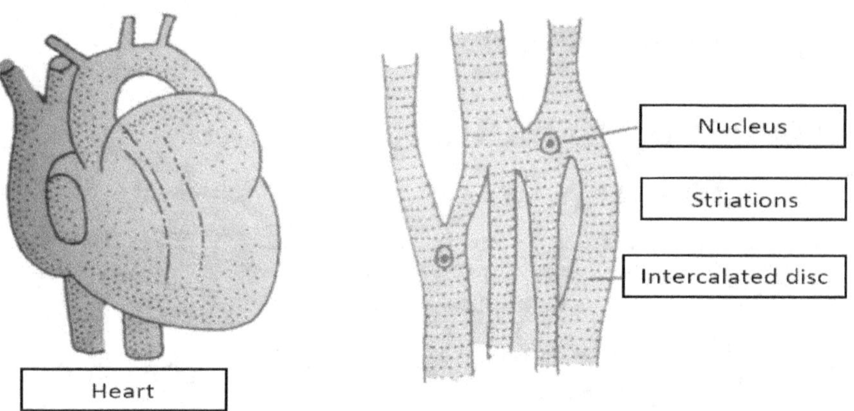

S. NO.	CHARACTERISTICS	CARDIAC MUSCLE
1.	Microscopic appearance and features	Branched cylindrical fibre with one centrally located nucleus; intercalated discs join neighbouring fibres; striated.
2.	Location	Heart
3.	Fibre diameter	Large (10-20 nm)
4.	Connective tissue components	Endomysium
5.	Fibre length	50-100 nm
6.	Contractile proteins organised into sarcomeres	Yes
7.	Sarcoplasmic reticulum	Some
8.	Transverse tubules present	Yes, aligned with each z disc.
9.	Junction between fibres	Intercalated discs, certain gap junction and desmosomes
10.	Auto rhythmicity	Yes
11.	Sources of calcium ion for contraction	Sarcoplasmic reticulum and interstitial fluid.
12.	Regular proteins for contraction	Troponin and tropomyosin
13.	Speed of contraction	Moderate
14.	Nervous control	Involuntary
15.	Contraction regulated by	Acetylcholine and norepinephrine released by autonomic motor neurons; several hormones.
16.	Capacity for regeneration	Limited, under certain conditions.

Observation: Cardiac tissue slides were studied using compound microscope

Result: The microscopic structure of cardiac muscle were studied and its structure is drawn.

Experiment No.: 5

Microscopic Examination of Smooth Muscles

Objective:	To study microscopic structure of smooth muscles using compound microscope
Equipment/ Glassware Required:	Charts /models/slides of smooth muscle / compound microscope

Principle

These are called smooth muscles because they are plain, non-striated, involuntary and unstriped muscles unlike cardiac and skeletal muscles. This gives smooth muscle the ability to contract for longer but at slower pace. Smooth muscles occur in the walls of hollow internal organs like alimentary canal, gall bladder, respiratory tract, uterus, urinary bladder, blood vessels, etc. Smooth muscle is almost everywhere in your body and aids in everything such as circulation, digestion, reproduction, respiration, etc. Unlike skeletal muscles, smooth muscles are not connected to bones.

Procedure

Collect the chart or tissue slide and observe the slides of smooth muscle under compound microscope for their structure and arrangement with respect to their function as follows:

1. Spindle shaped smooth muscle, thickest in middle and tapering at both ends
2. The location of single nucleus and its pattern
3. Characteristic presence of non-striated fibers
4. Place of junction between fibers
5. Un-branching pattern of smooth muscles
6. Draw the observation and label it

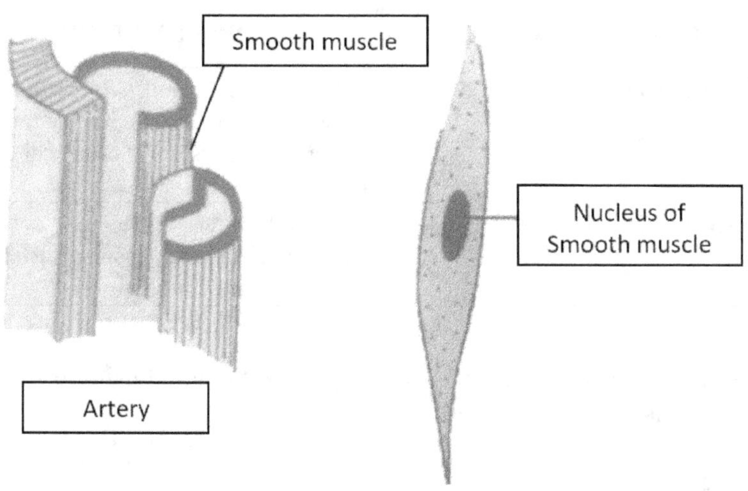

S. NO.	CHARACTERISTICS	OBSERVATION
1.	Microscopic appearance and features	Fibre is thickest in middle, tapered each end and has one centrally positioned nucleus not striated.
2.	Location	Walls of hollow viscera, airways, blood vessels, iris and ciliary body of eye, erector pili muscles of hair follicles,
3.	Fibre diameter	(3-8 nm)
4.	Connective tissue components	Endomysium
5.	Fibre length	30-200 nm
6.	Contractile proteins organised into sarcomeres	No
7.	Sarcoplasmic reticulum	Very little
8.	Transverse tubules present	No
9.	Junction between fibres	Gap junctions in visceral smooth muscle, none in multiunit smooth muscle.
10.	Auto rhythmicity	Yes, in visceral smooth muscle.
11.	Sources of calcium ion for contraction	Sarcoplasmic reticulum and interstitial fluid.
12.	Regular proteins for contraction	Calmodium and myosin light chain kinase.
13.	Speed of contraction	Slow
14.	Nervous control	Involuntary

Table contd…

S. NO.	CHARACTERISTICS	OBSERVATION
15.	Contraction regulated by	Acetylcholine and norepinephrine released by autonomic motor neurons; several hormones; local chemical charge, stretching.
16.	Capacity for regeneration	considerable via pericytes compared with other muscle tissue, but limited compared with epithelium.

Observation: Smooth muscle tissue slides were studied using microscope and diagram is drawn with label.

Result: The microscopic structure of smooth muscle were studied in detail.

Experiment No.: 6

Microscopic Examination of Skeletal Muscles

Objective:	To study the skeletal muscles with the help of compound microscope
Equipment/ Glassware Required:	Charts /models/slides of muscular tissues, compound microscope

Principle

These types of muscles are also called voluntary muscles because there is a conscious control over it. These muscles are attached to the bones through tendons and helps in movement of the skeleton therefore they are called as skeletal muscles. They are also referred to striated or stripped muscle because of the characteristic pattern of the cell which consist of the large number of muscle fibres. The entire muscle is covered in a connective tissue sheath called the 'epimysium' within the muscles the cells are collected into separate bundles called 'fascicles' and each fascicle is covered in its own connective tissue sheath called 'perimysium' and within the fascicles are the individual muscle cell. Each muscle grabbed into fine connective tissue layer called endomysium. Each of these connective tissue layers are inter-connected muscle fibres do not attach directly to the bones. But rather through specialized extensions of fibrous tissue covering in the form of 'tendons'. Tendons are often rope like structure but has a broad structure called aponeuroses. Fleshy part of the muscle called belly. The plasma membrane of muscle cell is called 'sarcolemma' and cytoplasm is called 'sarcoplasm'. Sarcoplasm contains a red coloured protein called myoglobin. When you observe at higher magnification sarcoplasm appears stuffed with little threads called 'myofibrils' a fluid filled system of membranous sacs called the 'sarcoplasmic reticulum' or SR encircles each myofibrils.

Procedure

Collect the chart or tissue slide and observe the slides of skeletal muscle under compound microscope for their structure and arrangement with respect to their function as follows:

1. Long cylindrical fibres enclosing sarcolemma
2. Recognize dark 'A' and light 'I' bands giving characteristic appearance of striated muscles
3. The location of nucleus and its pattern of arrangement
4. Observe epimysium, perimysium, endomysium and fascicles
5. Note arrangement of little threads myofibrils in sarcoplasm
6. Observe the belly
7. Identify the sarcoplasm appears red coloured due to presence of myoglobin
8. Draw the observation and label it

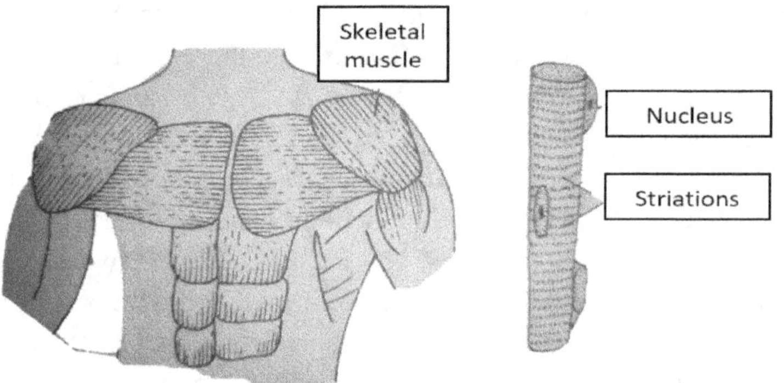

S. No.	Characteristics	Skeletal muscle
1.	Microscopic appearance and features	Long cylindrical fibre with many peripherally located nuclei; striated.
2.	Location	Most commonly attached by tendons to bones.
3.	Fibre diameter	Very large (10-100 nm)
4.	Connective tissue components	Endomysium, Perimysium, and epimysium
5.	Fibre length	100 nm - 300 nm

Table *contd...*

S. No.	Characteristics	Skeletal muscle
6.	Contractile proteins organised into sarcomeres	Yes
7.	Sarcoplasmic reticulum	Abundant
8.	Transverse tubules present	Yes, aligned with each A-I band junction.
9.	Junction between fibres	None
10.	Auto rhythmicity	No
11.	Sources of calcium ion for contraction	Sarcoplasmic reticulum
12.	Regular proteins for contraction	Troponin and tropomyosin
13.	Speed of contraction	Fast
14.	Nervous control	Voluntary
15.	Contraction regulated by	Acetylcholine released by somatic motor neurons.
16.	Capacity for regeneration	Limited, via satellite cells.

Observation: Anatomical and microscopic features of skeletal muscle are observed and noted.

Result: The structure and function of skeletal muscle were studied with the help of models, charts, and diagrams.

Experiment No.: 7

Microscopic Examination of Connective Tissue

Objective:	To study the structure and function of connective tissue with the help of compound microscope, chart and models
Equipment/ Glassware Required:	Charts /models/slides of connective tissue / compound microscope

Principle

Connective tissue connects and supports all other tissues hence called as connective tissue. It is one of the most widely distributed tissues in the body constituting about 30% of body composition. It performs various functions due to its different forms. It has majorly three different functions i.e. mechanical, nutritive and defensive. These functions can be explained based on the following;

1. It binds together, supports, and strengthens other body tissues

2. It protects and insulates internal organs

3. It serves as the major transport system within the body (blood, a fluid connective tissue)

4. It is the primary location of stored energy reserves (adipose, or fat, tissue)

5. It is the main source of immune responses

Procedure

Take the chart or observe the slides of different tissue under compound microscope and study their structure.

- Connective tissue consists of two basic elements: extracellular matrix and cells.

- A connective tissue's extracellular matrix is the material located between its widely spaced cells.

- The extracellular matrix consists of protein fibers and ground substance, the material between the cells and the fibers.
- The extracellular matrix is usually secreted by the connective tissue cells and determines the tissue's qualities.

Classification of Connective Tissues

I. Embryonic connective tissue

    A.   Mesenchyme

    B.   Mucous connective tissue

II. Mature connective tissue

    A. Loose connective tissue

        1. Areolar connective tissue

        2. Adipose tissue

        3. Reticular connective tissue

    B. Dense connective tissue

        1. Dense regular connective tissue

        2. Dense irregular connective tissue

        3. Elastic connective tissue

    C. Cartilage

        1. Hyaline cartilage

        2. Fibrocartilage

        3. Elastic cartilage

    D. Bone tissue

    E. Liquid connective tissue

        1. Blood tissue

        2. Lymph

I. Embryonic connective tissue

A. Mesenchyme

Description: Consists of irregularly shaped mesenchymal cells embedded in a semifluid ground substance that contains reticular fibres.

Location: Under skin and along developing bones of embryo; some mesenchymal cells are found in adult connective tissue, especially along blood vessels.

Function: Forms all other types of connective tissue

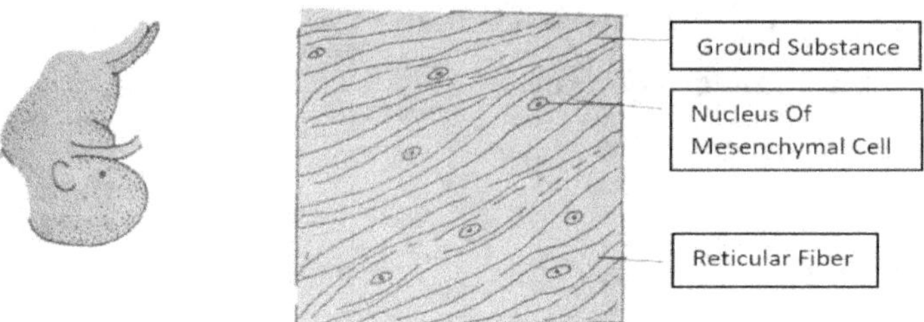

B. Mucous connective tissue

Description: Consists of widely scattered fibroblasts embedded in a viscous, jellylike ground substance that contains fine collagen fibers.

Location: Umbilical cord of foetus.

Function: Support.

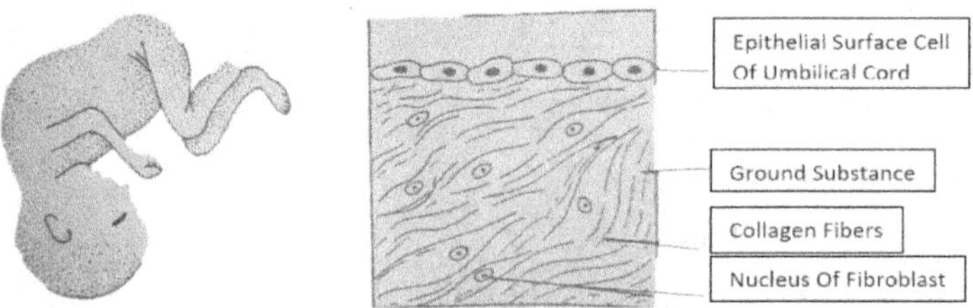

II. Mature connective tissue

A. Loose connective tissue

1. Areolar connective tissue

Description: Consists of fibres (collagen, elastic, and reticular) and several kinds of cells (fibroblasts, macrophages, plasma cells, adipocytes, and mast cells) embedded in a semifluid ground substance.

Location: Subcutaneous layer deep to skin; papillary (superficial) region of dermis of skin; lamina propria of mucous membranes; and around blood vessels, nerves, and body organs.

Function: Strength, elasticity, and support.

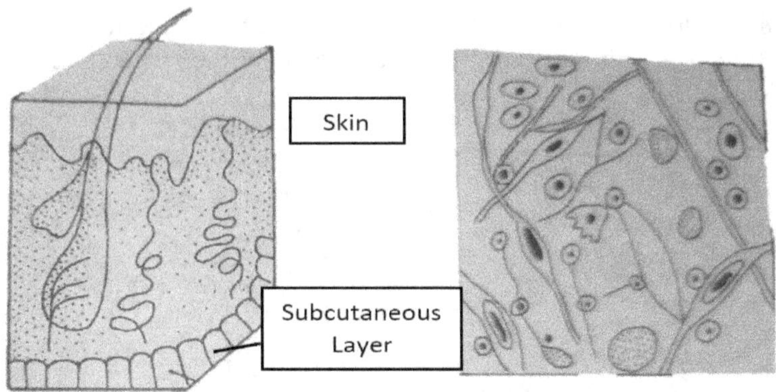

2. Adipose tissue

Description: Consists of adipocytes, cells specialized to store triglycerides (fats) as a large centrally located droplet; nucleus and cytoplasm are peripherally located.

Location: Subcutaneous layer deep to skin, around heart and kidneys, yellow bone marrow, and padding around joints and behind eyeball in eye socket.

Function: Reduces heat loss through skin, serves as an energy reserve, supports, and protects. In newborns, brown adipose tissue generates considerable heat that helps maintain proper body temperature.

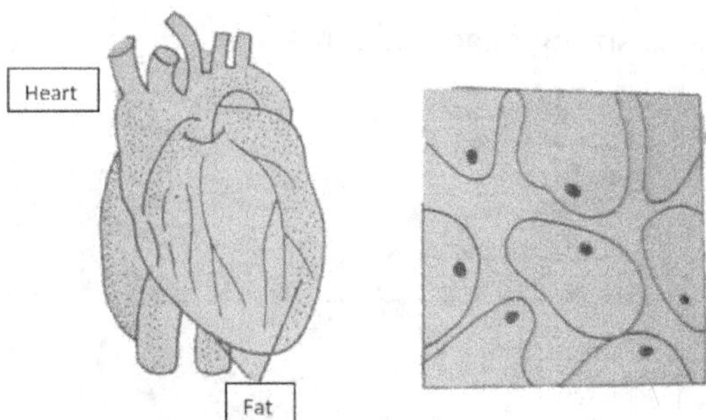

3. Reticular connective tissue

Description: A network of interlacing reticular fibers and reticular cells.

Location: Stroma (supporting framework) of liver, spleen, lymph nodes; red bone marrow, which gives rise to blood cells; reticular lamina of the basement membrane; and around blood vessels and muscles.

Function: Forms stroma of organs; binds together smooth muscle tissue cells; filters and removes worn-out blood cells in the spleen and microbes in lymph nodes.

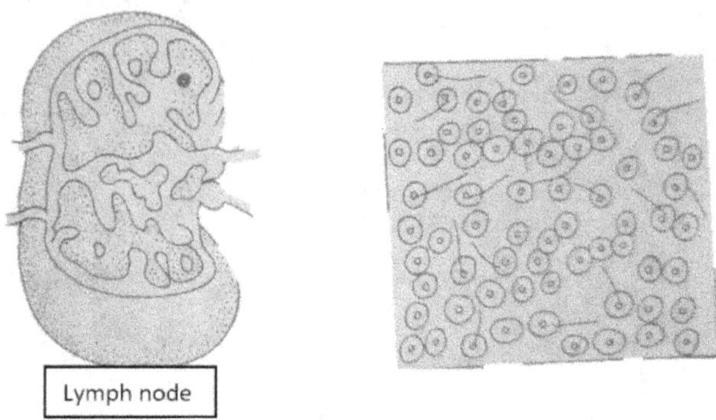

B. Dense connective tissue

1. Dense regular connective tissue

Description: Extracellular matrix looks shiny white; consists mainly of collagen fibers regularly arranged in bundles; fibroblasts present in rows between bundles.

Location: Forms tendons (attach muscle to bone), most ligaments (attach bone to bone), and aponeuroses (sheet like tendons that attach muscle to muscle or muscle to bone).

Function: Provides strong attachment between various structures.

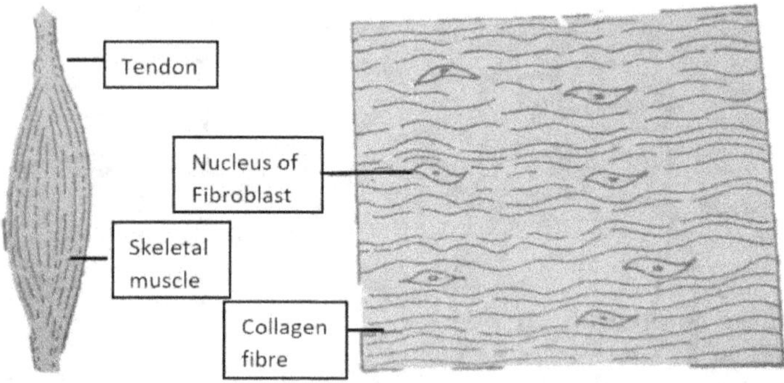

2. Dense irregular connective tissue

Description: Consists predominantly of collagen fibers randomly arranged and a few fibroblasts.

Location: Fasciae (tissue beneath skin and around muscles and other organs), reticular (deeper) region of dermis of skin, periosteum of bone, perichondrium of cartilage, joint capsules, membrane capsules around various organs (kidneys, liver, testes, lymph nodes), pericardium of the heart, and heart valves.

Function: Provides strength.

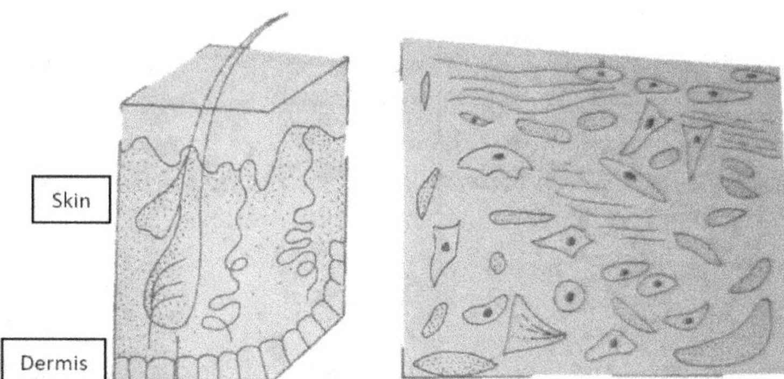

3. Elastic connective tissue

Description: Consists predominantly of freely branching elastic fibers; fibroblasts are present in spaces between fibers.

Location: Lung tissue, walls of elastic arteries, trachea, bronchial tubes, true vocal cords, suspensory ligament of penis, and some ligaments between vertebrae.

Function: Allows stretching of various organs.

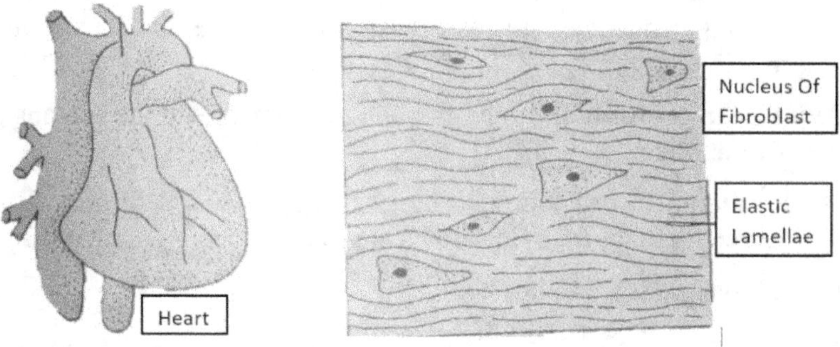

C. Cartilage

1. Hyaline cartilage

Description: Consists of a bluish-white, shiny ground substance with thin, fine collagen fibers and many chondrocytes; most abundant type of cartilage.

Location: Ends of long bones, anterior ends of ribs, nose, parts of larynx, trachea, bronchi, bronchial tubes, and embryonic and fetal skeleton.

Function: Provides smooth surfaces for movement at joints, as well as flexibility and support.

2. Fibrocartilage

Description: Consists of chondrocytes scattered among thick bundles of collagen fibers within the extracellular matrix.

Location: Pubic symphysis (point where hip bones join anteriorly), intervertebral discs (discs between vertebrae), menisci (cartilage pads) of knee, and portions of tendons that insert into cartilage.

Function: Support and fusion

3. Elastic cartilage

Description: Consists of chondrocytes located in a threadlike network of elastic fibers within the extracellular matrix.

Location: Lid on top of larynx (epiglottis), part of external ear (auricle), and auditory (eustachian) tubes.

Function: Gives support and maintains shape.

D. Bone tissue

Description: Compact bone tissue consists of osteons (haversian systems) that contain lamellae, lacunae, osteocytes, canaliculi, and central (haversian) canals. By contrast, spongy bone tissue, it consists of thin columns called trabeculae; spaces between trabeculae are filled with red bone marrow.

Location: Both compact and spongy bone tissue make up the various parts of bones of the body.

Function: Support, protection, storage; houses blood-forming tissue; serves as levers that act with muscle tissue to enable movement.

E. Liquid Connective Tissue

1. Blood

Description: Blood constitutes about 8% of total body weight. It is composed of 55% plasma and 45% cells. The cells include red blood corpuscles (RBC), White blood cells (WBC) and platelets. Further WBCs are classified as granulocytes for Neutrophils, Eosinophils and Basophils; and agranulocytes i.e. lymphocytes and monocytes.

Location: It circulates in artery and vein blood vessels with the help of pumping action of heart and capillary movement.

Function: It plays vital role in carrying oxygen, nutrients, and hormones to cells. It also helps in maintaining body homeostasis and body defensive mechanism against pathogens.

2. Lymph

Description: Lymph is derived from interstitial fluid containing lymph plasma similar to blood plasma. However the glucose, lipid and protein concentration is higher than blood.

Location: It is circulated in lymph capillaries, lymph channels, lymph nodes and lymph trunks.

Function: It is involved in transportation of oxygen, nutrients, hormones along with removal of metabolic waste from the cells. Helps in maintaining the composition and volume of blood. It also helps in absorption of fat soluble vitamins. It protects the body from invasion of microbes and other substance.

Observation: The macroscopic and microscopic features of various connective tissues are studied.

Result: The microscopic structure of various connective tissues were studied and diagrams drawn.

Experiment No.: 8

Microscopic Examination of Nervous Tissue

Objective:	To study the structure and function of nervous tissue with the help of compound microscope, chart and models
Equipment/ Glassware Required:	Charts /models/slides of connective tissue / compound microscope

Principle

Nervous tissue is one of the complex tissue in the body, composed of densely packed interconnected neurons (nerve cells). It is specialized in communication between various parts of body. It controls and coordinate different body functions through exhibiting sensitivity to various types of stimuli into nerve impulses (action potential) and conduct nerve impulses to other neurons, muscle fibres, or glands.

Identification features of nervous tissue include a large cell body (cyton), with a prominent nucleus. Cyton has cytoplasmic projections called dendrites, one of the projection is long and is called axon. A myelin sheath is present over the myelinated nerve fibre. A membrane neurolemma surrounds the myelin sheath.

Neuroglia or Glia cells are supporting and packing cells found in brain, spinal cord and ganglia. They do not generate and conduct nerve impulse and being non-nervous cell perform important protection from injuries and other damages and also helps the nerve cells by providing nutrition.

Dendrite projection from cell body mainly consists of Nissl's granules and mitrochondria involved in conducting nerve impulse towards the body. Axon is the longer single projection without Nissl's granules and cylindrical projection of uniform diameter and conducts nerve impulses away from the body.

Procedure

Take the chart or observe the slides of different tissue under compound microscope and study their structure.

- The large body containing nucleus is called cell body.
- Shorter projections from cell body are dendrites
- Longer projection from cell body is axon
- Draw the diagram of observation and label it

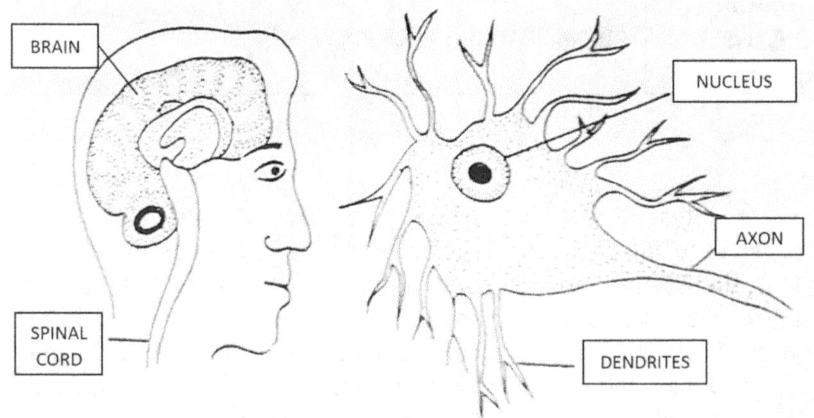

Observation: Characteristic features of nervous tissues are studied with the help of compound microscope and pre-prepared permanent slides.

Result: Microscopic features of nervous tissue are studied and diagrams are drawn.

Experiment No.: 9

Study of Human Skeleton-Axial Skeleton

Objective:	To study the general features of axial skeletal system
Equipment/ Glassware Required:	Skeletal system model or chart

Principle

The skeletal system is defined as bony framework of the body to support and protect the soft and vital parts present inside the body. It is composed of bones, their cartilages, along with ligaments and tendons. Bones come in a variety of shapes and sizes and have a complex internal and external structure. They are lightweight yet strong and hard, and serve multiple functions. Depending upon the location, function and supportive features it could be divided into 1. Axial skeleton and 2. Appendicular skeleton. The functions of the skeletal system are to:

a) Support & protect soft tissue &vital organs

b) Give attachment to skeletal muscles.

c) Synthesize blood cells in the bone marrow.

d) Store mineral salts like phosphorus & calcium

The Axial skeleton system it occupies body's main longitudinal axis, run through the centre of gravity therefore called as axial skeleton. It includes skull, vertebral column, ribs and sternum. Total number of bones present in axial skeleton, 80 in adults and 87 in children.

The vertebral column, also known as the spinal column, is the central axis of the skeleton in all vertebrates. The vertebral column provides attachments to muscles, supports the trunk, protects the spinal cord and nerve roots and serves as a site for haemopoiesis. The sternum or breastbone is a long flat bone located in the central part of the chest. It connects to the ribs via cartilage and forms the front of the rib cage, thus helping to protect the heart, lungs, and major blood vessels from injury. The ribs are the bony framework of the thoracic cavity. The ribs form the main structure of the thoracic cage protecting the thoracic organs; however, their main function is to help in respiration.

Procedure

Collect model or chart of the skeletal system and identify the parts of a long bone, number, and types of bones present in the axial skeletal system.

Comparison of Bones of adult axial and appendicular skeleton system	
Axial skeleton (80 bones) **Skull** Cranium=8 Face=14 **Hyoid**=1 **Auditory Ossicles**=6	**Appendicular skeleton (126 bones)** **Pectoral girdles** clavical=2, scapula=2
	Upper limbs (extremities) humerus=2, ulna=2, radius=2, carpals=16, metacarpals=10 phalanges=28
Vertebral column=26	**Pelvic girdles** hip, pelvic or coxal bone=2
Thorax Sternum=1 Ribs=24	**Lower limbs (extremities)** Femur=2 patella=2 fibula=2 tibia=2 tarsal=14 metatarsals=10 Phalanges=28

Different bones of axial skeletal system:

1. **Skull:** It is made up of eight cranium, fourteen of facial bones, one hyoid bone, and six auditory ossicles.

2. **Hyoid bone:** The hyoid bone is U- shaped. It is a unique component of the axial skeleton because it does not articulate with any other bone. It supports the tongue providing attachment sites for some tongue muscles & muscles of the neck.

3. **Vertebral column:** It is also called spine or backbone, makeup about two-fifth of our total height. The spinal cord that it surrounds and protects consists of nervous & connective tissue.

4. **Sternum:** It is also called breastbone. It is a flat, narrow bone located in the center of the anterior thoracic wall that measures about 15 cm in length.

5. **Ribs:** Twelve pairs of ribs give structural support to the sides of the thoracic cavity. The ribs increase in length from first to seventh, then decrease to twelfth rib.

6. **Clavicle:** It is also called collar bone. It is a long & curved bone. It forms the anterior part of the shoulder girdle. It contains a shaft, two ends & four borders.

7. **Scapula:** Scapula or shoulder blade is a large, flat bone situated in the superior part of the posterior thorax between the levels of the second & seventh ribs.

8. **Humerus:** The humerus or arm bone is the longest &largest bone of the upper limb.

9. **Ulna:** The ulna is located on the medial aspect of the forearm & is longer than the radius. It provides attachment for the ulnar collateral ligament to the wrist.

10. **Radius:** It is located on the lateral aspect of the forearm. It articulates with three bones of the wrist- the lunate, the scaphoid & the triquetrum to form the wrist joint.

11. **Carpals:** It is the proximal region of the hand & consists of eight small bones, the carpals, joined to one another by ligaments.

12. **Metacarpals:** Palms is the intermediate region of the hand & consist of five bones called metacarpals.

13. **Phalanges:** Bone of the digits, make up the distal part of the hand. There are 14 phalanges in the five digits of each hand & like the metacarpals.

14. **Pelvic girdle:** It is also called coxal bones. The bony pelvis provides strong & stable support for the vertebral column & pelvic organs.

15. **Femur:** It is the longest, heaviest & strongest bone in the body. Its proximal end articulates with the acetabulum of the hip bone. It serves as attachment points for the tendons of several thigh muscles.

16. **Patella:** It is a small, triangular bone located anterior to the knee joint. It protects the knee joint.

17. **Tibia and fibula:** The tibia or shin bone is the larger, medial, weight-bearing bone of the leg. It articulates at its proximal end with the femur & fibula. The fibula is parallel & lateral to the tibia but it is considerably smaller.

18. **Tarsal and metatarsals:** It is the proximal region of the foot & consists of 7 tarsal bones. The calcaneus is the largest & strongest tarsal bone. The metatarsal, the intermediate region of the foot consists of five metatarsal bones numbered from the medial to lateral.

19. **Phalanges:** It comprises the distal component of the foot & resembles those at the hand both in number & arrangement

The Skull

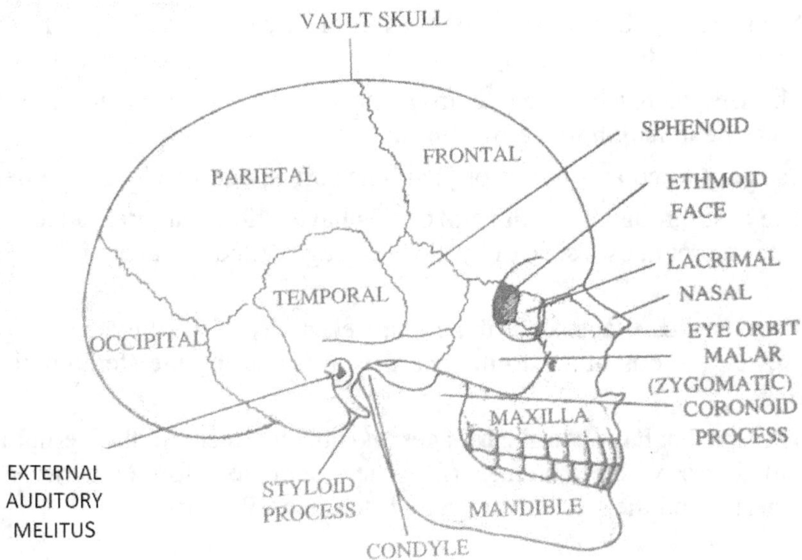

The sternum, or breastbone

- It is a flat, narrow bone located in the center of the anterior thoracic wall that measures about 15 cm. in length

- It consists of three parts. The superior part is the manubrium; the middle and largest part is the body; and the inferior, smallest part is the xiphoid process.

- The segments of the sternum typically fuse by age 25, and the points of fusion are marked by transverse ridges.

- The junction of the manubrium and body forms the sternal angle. The manubrium has a depression on its superior surface, the suprasternal notch.

- Lateral to the suprasternal notch are clavicular notches that articulate with the medial ends of the clavicles to form the sternoclavicular joints. The manubrium also articulates with the costal cartilages of the first and second ribs.

- The body of the sternum articulates directly or indirectly with the costal cartilages of the second through tenth ribs.

- The xiphoid process consists of hyaline cartilage during infancy and childhood and does not completely ossify until about age 40. No ribs are attached to it, but the xiphoid process provides attachment for some abdominal muscles.

Twelve pairs of ribs

- Numbered 1-12 from superior to inferior, give structural support to the sides of the thoracic cavity.

- The ribs increase in length from the first through seventh, and then decrease in length to the twelfth rib.

- Each rib articulates posteriorly with its corresponding thoracic vertebra.

- The first through seventh pairs of ribs have a direct anterior attachment to the sternum by a strip of hyaline cartilage called costal cartilage (cost-rib).

- The costal cartilages contribute to the elasticity of the thoracic cage and prevent various blows to the chest from fracturing the sternum and/or ribs.

- The ribs that have costal cartilages and attach directly to the sternum are called true (vertebra-sternal) ribs. The articulations formed between the true ribs and the sternum are called sternocostal joints.

- The remaining five pairs of ribs are termed false ribs because their costal cartilages either attach indirectly to the sternum or do not attach to the sternum at all.

- The cartilages of the eighth, ninth, and tenth pairs of ribs attach to one another and then to the cartilages of the seventh pair of ribs. These false ribs are called vertebra-chondral ribs.

- The eleventh and twelfth pairs of ribs are false ribs designated as floating (vertebral) ribs because the costal cartilage at their anterior ends does not attach to the sternum at all. These ribs attach only posteriorly to the thoracic vertebrae.

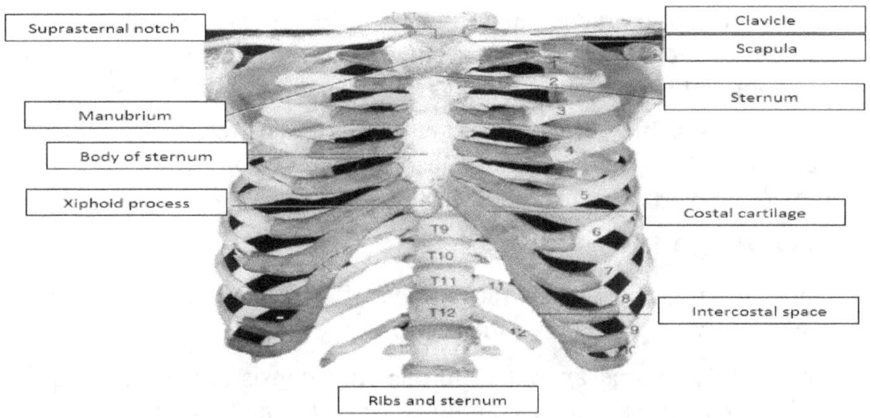

The vertebral column

- Also called the spine or backbone,
- Makes up about two-fifths of height and is composed of a series of bones called vertebrae.
- The vertebral column, the sternum, and the ribs form the skeleton of the trunk of the body.
- At about 71cm in an average adult male and about 61cm in an average adult female, the vertebral column functions as a strong, flexible rod with elements that can move forward, backward, and sideways, and rotate.
- In addition to enclosing and protecting the spinal cord, it supports the head, and serves as a point of attachment for the ribs, pelvic girdle, and muscles of the back.

- The total number of vertebrae during early development is 33, as child grows, several vertebrae in the sacral and coccygeal regions fuse. As a result, the adult vertebral column, also called the spinal column, typically contains 26 vertebrae. These are distributed as follows:

  - 7 cervical vertebrae are in the neck region

  - 12 thoracic vertebrae are posterior to the thoracic cavity

  - 5 lumbar vertebrae support the lower back

  - 1 sacrum consists of five fused sacral vertebrae

  - 1 coccyx usually consists of four fused coccygeal vertebrae.

- The cervical, thoracic, and lumbar vertebrae are movable, but the sacrum and coccyx are not. When viewed from the side, the adult vertebral column shows four slight bends called normal curves.

- The curves of the vertebral column increase its strength, help maintain balance in the upright position, absorb shocks during walking, and help protect the vertebrae from the fracture.

Intervertebral Discs

- They are found between the bodies of adjacent vertebrae from the second cervical vertebra to the sacrum.

- Each disc contains an outer fibrous ring consisting of fibrocartilage called the annulus fibrosus (annulus=ring like) and an inner soft, pulpy, highly elastic substance called the nucleus pulposus (pulposus= pulplike).

- The disk forms the strong joints, permit various movements of the vertebral column, and absorb vertical shock.

Parts of a Typical vertebra

- **The body**: It is thick, disc-shaped anterior portion, is the weight bearing part of a vertebra. Its superior and inferior surfaces are roughened for the attachment of cartilaginous intervertebral discs. The anterior and lateral surfaces contain nutrient foramina, openings through which blood vessels deliver nutrients and oxygen and remove carbon dioxide and wastes from the bone tissue.

- **The vertebral (neural) arch**: two short, thick processes, the pedicles, posteriorly from the vertebral body to unite with the flat laminae, to form the vertebral arch. The vertebral arch extends posteriorly from the body of the vertebra; together the body of the vertebrae and the vertebral arch surrounds the spinal cord by forming the vertebral foramen.

The vertebral foramen contains the spinal cord, adipose tissue areolar connective tissue, and blood vessels. Collectively, the vertebral foramina of all vertebrae form the vertebral (spinal cavity). The pedicles exhibit superior and inferior indentations called vertebral notches. When the vertebral notches are stacked on top of one another, they form an opening between adjoining vertebrae on both sides of the column. Each opening, called an intervertebral foramen, permits the passage of a single spinal nerve that passes to a specific region of the body.

Processes

- Seven processes arise from the vertebral arch. At the point where a lamina and pedicle join, a transverse process extends laterally on each side. A single spinous process projects posteriorly from the junction of the laminae. These three processes serve as points of attachment for muscles.

- The remaining four processes form joints with other vertebrae above or below. The two superior articular processes of a vertebra articulate with the two inferior articular processes of the vertebra immediately above them. In turn, the two inferior articular processes of that vertebra immediately below them, and so on. The articulating surfaces of the articular processes, which are referred to as facets, are covered with the hyaline cartilage. The articulations formed between the bodies and articular facets of successive vertebrae are termed intervertebral joints.

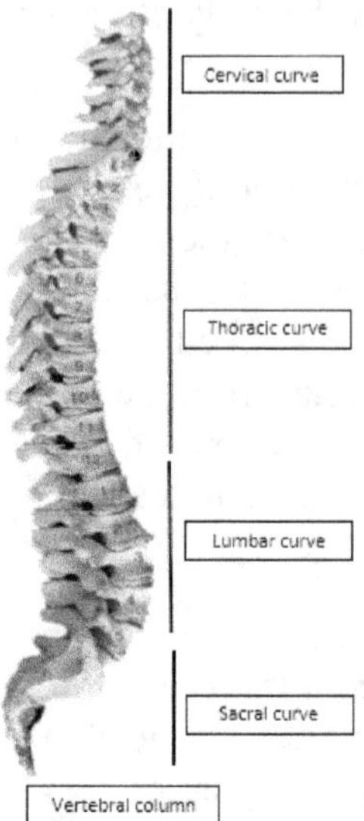

Observation: The axial bones and joints are studied with the help of charts and models

Result: Human axial skeletal system were studied, diagram drawn and labeled.

Experiment No.: 10

Study of Human Skeleton-Appendicular Skeleton

Objective:	To study appendicular skeletal system using charts or models
Equipment/ Glassware Required:	Model or Chart of appendicular skeletal system

Principle

The appendages of axial skeleton system are called appendicular skeleton system consisting of bones which helps in movement of body. These bones are either the part of pelvic girdle (hip) or pectoral girdle (shoulder). The primary role of pelvic girdle is to support the weight of the upper body when sitting and to transfer this weight to the lower limbs when standing. It serves as an attachment point for trunk and lower limb muscles, and also protects the internal pelvic organs. The lower limb consists of four major parts: a girdle formed by the hip bones, the thigh, the leg, and the foot. It is specialized for the support of weight, adaptation to gravity, and locomotion.

Pectoral girdle or shoulder girdle consist of the following parts:

The human body has two pectoral or shoulder girdles that attaches the bones of the upper limbs to the axial skeleton. Scapula, clavicle, one each and bones of upper limb. The upper limb consists of one each of humerus, radius, ulna and 8 carpal bones, 5 metacarpal bones, and 14 phalanges. The clavicle (also called collar bone) is the anterior bone and articulates with the manubrium of the sternum at the sternoclavicular joint. The scapula articulates with the clavicle at the acromioclavicular joint and with the humerus at the glenohumeral joint.

Pectoral girdles do not articulate with the vertebral column and are held in position by muscular attachments.

Procedure

Collect model or chart of the appendicular system and then study and identify their parts.

Clavicle

a) Each slender, s-shaped clavicle or collar bone, lies horizontally across the anterior part of the thorax superior to the first rib

b) It has a shaft and two ends called as acrominal and sternal ends

c) The acrominal end is flat and forms acrominal joint with acrominal process of the scapula.

d) The clavicle transmits mechanical force from the upper limb to the trunk via the clavicular ligaments

e) The clavicle is one of the most frequently broken bone in the body

f) The clavicle keeps the shoulder away from the trunk and thereby enabling the upper limb to swing clear of the trunk

Scapula

a) Each scapula or shoulder blade is a large, triangular, flat bone situated in the superior part of the posterior thorax between the levels of second and seventh ribs

b) The thin edges of the scapula closer to the vertebral column is called the medial border

c) The thick edge of the scapula closer to the arm is called the lateral border

d) The medial and lateral borders join at the inferior

e) The superior edges of the scapula, called the superior border joins the medial border at the superior angle

f) The superior angle is the point at which the superior and the medial border of the scapula meet

g) On the anterior surface of the scapula is a slightly hollowed out area called the subscapular

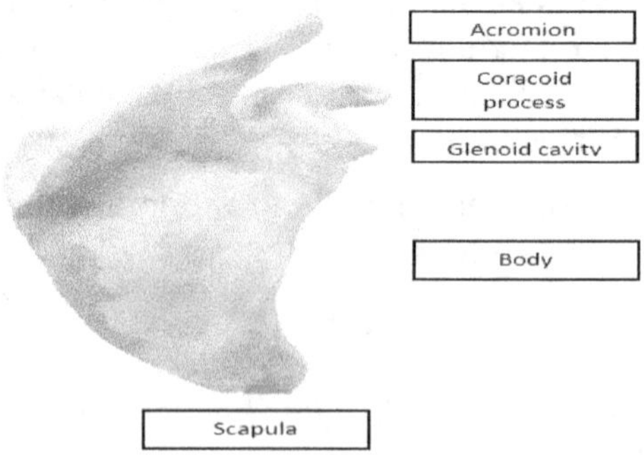

Upper limb: Each upper limb has 30 bones in three locations: -

The humerus in the arm, the ulna and radius in the forearm, 8 carpals in the wrist (carpus), the 5 metacarpals in the metacarpus (palm) and 14 phalanges (bones of the digits) in the hand.

Humerus

a) The humerus or arm bone, is the longest and largest bone of the upper limb

b) It articulates proximally with the scapula and distally at the elbow with two bones, the ulna and radius

c) The body or shaft of the humerus is roughly cylindrical at its proximal end

d) The proximal end consists of head, neck, greater tubercle and lesser tubercle

e) On the anterior aspect of the bone and immediately above the articular surface there is a deep fossa called olecranon fossa. This gives attachment to muscles and ligaments.

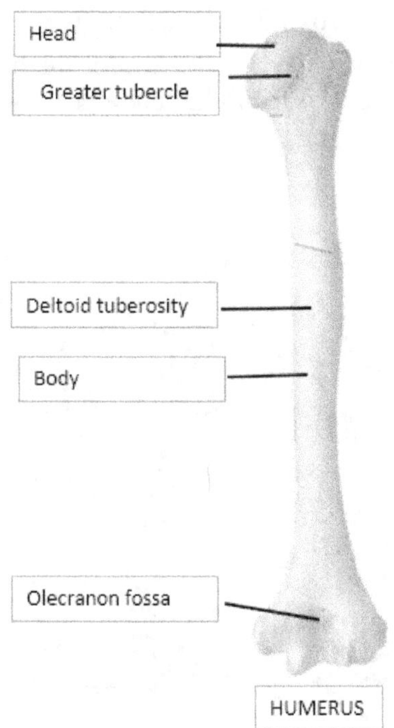

Ulna

a) The ulna is located on the medial aspect of foreman and is longer than the radius

b) This bone is long

c) It presents proximal end, shaft, distal end and the olecranon process forms the point of elbow and fits into the olecranon.

d) The distal end of the ulna consists of a head that is separated from the wrist by a disc of fibrocartilage

e) A styloid process is located on the posterior side of the ulnas distal end

f) It provides attachment for the ulna collateral ligament to the wrist.

Radius

a) The radius is located on the lateral aspect (thumb side) of the forearm

b) The proximal end of the radius has a disc-shaped head that articulates with the capitulum of the humerus and radial notch of the ulna

c) The distal end of the bones is expanded

d) The shaft of the radius widens to form a styloid- process on the lateral side which can be felt proximal to the thumb

e) The styloid process provides attachment for the brachioradialis muscle and for the attachment of the radial collateral ligaments to the wrist.

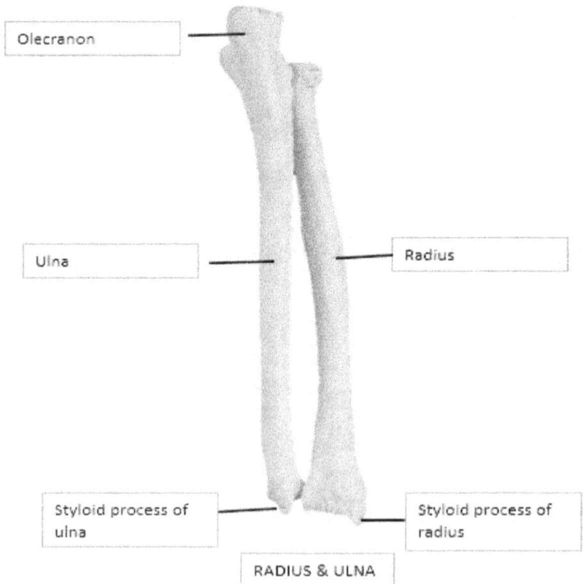

Carpals

a) The carpus (wrist) is the proximal region of the hand and consists of 8 small bones, joined to one another by ligaments

b) Eight carpals are arranged in two transverse rows of four bones each Scaphoid, innate, triquetrum, pisiform, trapezium, trapezoid, hamate, capital

c) These are closely fitted together and held in position which allows a certain amount of movement

Metacarpals

a) These are five in number and they form the structure of the palm of the hand

b) The proximal end of metacarpals articulated with the carpal and distal with phalanges

Phalanges

a) These are 14 in numbers

b) These are arranged 3 in each finger and 2 in each thumb

c) The thumb has no middle phalanges

d) Joints between phalanges are called interphalangeal joints

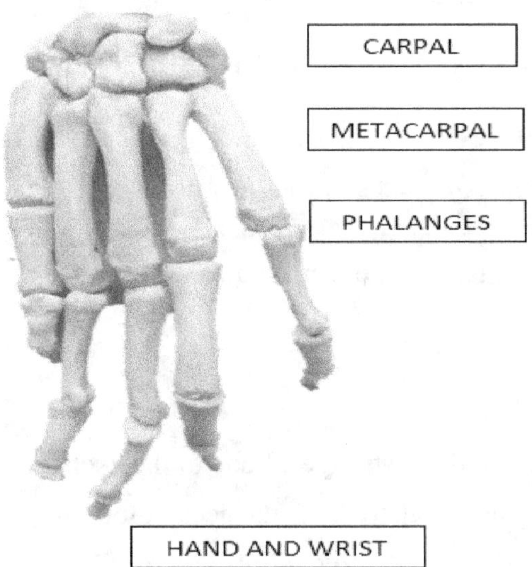

Pelvic (hip) girdle

a) The pelvic girdle consists of the two hip bones also called coxal or pelvic bones

b) The hip bones unite anteriorly at a joint called the pubic symphysis

c) They unite posteriorly with the sacrum at the sacroiliac joints

d) The pelvic girdle of the bony pelvis also connects the bones of the lower limbs to axial skeleton

e) Each of the two hip bones of a newborn consists of three bones separated by cartilage; a superior ilium, an inferior and anterior pubis and an inferior and posterior ischium

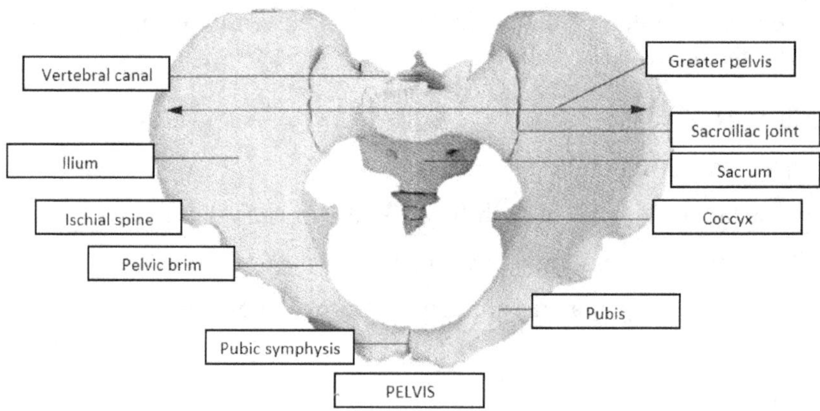

Lower limbs bones

Each lower limb has 30 bones in four locations

The femur in the thigh, the patella (knee cap), the tibia and fibula in the leg, the 7 tarsals in the tarsus, the 5 metatarsals in the metatarsus, and the 14 phalanges

Femur

a) It is the thigh bone

b) It is the longest and the strongest bone of the skeleton

c) Its proximal end articulates with the acetabulum of the hip bone

d) Its distal end articulates with the tibia and patella

e) Greater trochanter which is on the outer side where the neck joins the shaft

f) Lesser trochanter which is on the inner side where again the neck joins the shaft

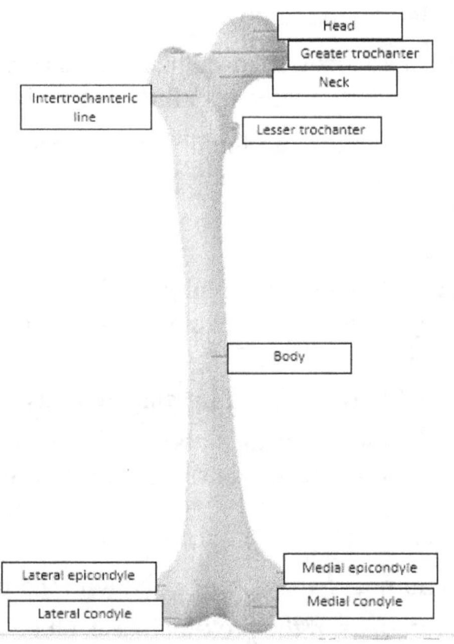

Patella

a) The patella or kneecap is a small, triangular bone located anterior to the knee joint

b) The posterior surface contains two articular faces, one for the medial condyle of the femur and another for the lateral condyle of the femur

c) The patella increases the leverage of the tendon of the quadriceps femories muscles, maintains the position of the tendon when the knee is bent and protect the knee joint

Tibia

a) It is the innermost bone of the leg

b) It is a long bone containing two extremity (upper and lower) and a shaft

c) The tibia articulates at its proximal end with the femur and fibula and its distal end with the fibula and the talus bone of the ankle

d) The proximal end of the tibia is expanded into a lateral condyle and a medial condyle

e) Of the long bone of the body, the tibia is the most frequently fractured and is also the most frequent site of an open fracture.

Fibula

a) It is parallel and lateral to the tibia, but it is considerably smaller

b) The distal end is more arrowhead shaped and has a projection called the lateral malleolus that articulates with the talus of the ankle

c) The fibula also articulates with the tibia at the fibular notch to form the distal tibiofibular joint

Tarsal

a) The tarsus(ankle) is the proximal region of the foot and consist of seven tarsal bones, they include following bones: - calcaneus-1, talus-1, navicula-1, cuboid-1, cuniform-3

b) Joints between tarsal bones called intertarsal joints

c) During walking the talus transmits about half the weight of the body to the calcaneus, the remainder is transmitted to the other tarsal bone

Metatarsals

a) They are five in numbers, they correspond with the five toes

b) Each metatarsal consists of the proximal base, an intermediate shaft and a distal head

c) The first metatarsal is thicker than the other because it bears more weight

Phalanges

The phalanges comprise the distal component of the foot and resemble those of the hand both in number and arrangement. The toes are numbered I to V beginning with the great toe, from medial to lateral. Each phalanx consists of a proximal base, an intermediate shaft, and a distal head. They are 14 bones, 2 for the first toe and 3 for the rest. All of these are long bones. Joints between phalanges of the foot, like those of the hands are called interphalangeal joints.

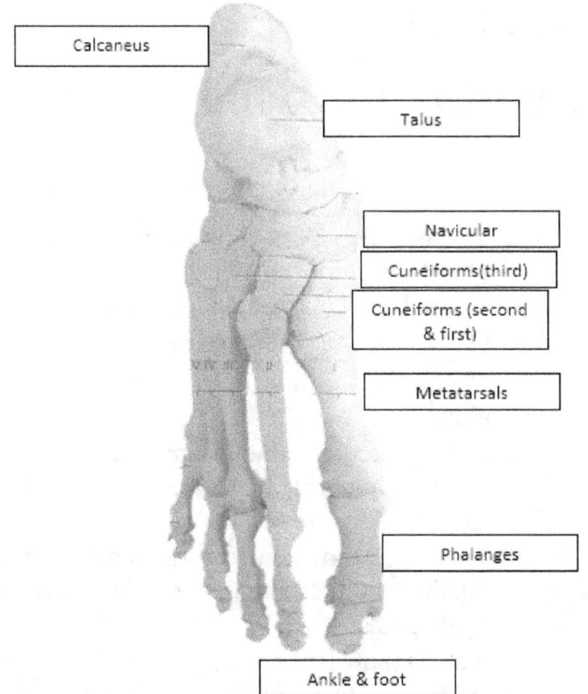

Observation: The appendicular skeletal system were studied and identified the parts using charts and models.

Result: Human appendicular-skeletal system were studied and diagrams are drawn with proper label.

Experiment No.: 11

Determination of Blood Group

Objective:	To determine the blood group of our own blood
Equipment / Glassware Required:	1. Microscope, glass dropper with a long nozzle, sterile blood lancet or needle, sterile cotton/ gauze swabs, alcohol, 5ml test tube, tooth picks. 2. Clean, dry microscope slides.
Chemicals Required:	1. 1% sodium citrate in normal saline (or normal saline alone) 2. Anti-A serum: contains monoclonal anti-A antibodies (against human); these are also called anti-A or alpha agglutinins. 3. Anti-B serum: contains monoclonal anti-B antibodies (against human); these are also called anti-B or beta agglutinins. 4. Anti-D (anti-Rh) serum: contain monoclonal anti-Rh (D) antibodies (against human). These antibodies are also called anti-D agglutinins. These antisera are available commercially. For a quick identification, the anti-A serum is tinted blue, anti-B serum yellow, while the anti-D serum is colorless.

Principle

According to the ABO system of blood group they are divided into four groups A, B, AB and O. The surface of red cell membrane contains a variety of genetically determined antigens, called agglutinogens, while the plasma contains antibodies (agglutinins). To determine the blood group of a person, his/her red cells are made to react with commercially available antisera containing known agglutinins.

For the determination of the blood group stock anti-sera A & B is required. These antisera have no agglutinogens but contain only the agglutinogens of the corresponding group (Stock Antisera A has 'a' agglutinin (antibody) and stock anti-sera B has 'b' agglutinin (antibody))

Blood Group	Antigen
A	Has only A antigen on red cells
B	Has only B antigen on red cells
AB	Has both A and B antigens on red cells
O	Has neither A nor B antigens on red cells

Compatible Blood Type Donors		
Blood Type	**Donate Blood To**	**Receive Blood From**
A+	A+, AB+	A+, A-, O+, OO
O+	O+, A+, B+, AB+	O+, O-
B+	B+, AB+	B+, B-, O+, O-
AB+	AB+	Everyone
A-	A+, A-, AB+, AB-	A-, O-
O-	Everyone	O-
B-	B+, B-, AB+, AB-	B-, O-
AB-	AB+, AB-	AB-, A-, B-, O-

Possible Blood Group of Child according to blood group of parents

Parent 1	AB	AB	AB	AB	B	A	A	O	O	O
Parent 2	AB	B	A	O	B	B	A	B	A	O
O	X	X	X	X	√	√	√	√	√	√
A	√	√	√	√	X	√	√	X	√	X
B	√	√	√	√	√	√	X	√	X	X
AB	√	√	√	X	X	√	X	X	X	X

Procedure

- Set the table with all the materials required
- Sterilize your finger tip with alcohol swab from where a drop of blood to be taken
- Gently rub the fingertip to improve blood circulation
- Take one drop of stock anti-A serum one end, stock anti-B serum in the middle of slide and and anti-D serum on another end of a slide.
- Prick the site with sterile needle or lancet.
- Press the fingertip to ooze sufficient blood required for all three ends of the slide.
- Add a very small drop of your own blood to all of them, and wait for 8-10 minutes, then inspect the 3 antisera -red cell mixture with the naked eye to see whether agglutination (clumping and hemolysis of red cells) has taken place or not.
- **Caution**
  - Do not interchange the droppers provided with antisera bottles.
  - Do not share/exchange needles and lancet
  - Do not reuse cotton swab, needle and lancet
  - Avoid pricking your finger if you have previous history of bleeding disorder
  - Dispose off used cotton swab, needle and lancets only in designated areas or biological waste disposal (yellow) boxes
  - Slides must be kept in plane horizontal area to avoid mixing of samples

Observation: The principle and procedure of blood group determination by antigen antibody was studied and following reaction between antigen and antibodies were observed:

1. If clumping occurs with anti-A serum (Blue bottle) only – Blood is of group A

2. If clumping occurs with anti-B serum (Yellow bottle) only – Blood is of group B

3. If clumping occurs with both anti-A serum and anti-B serum – Blood is of group AB

4. If no clumping occurred with anti-A serum and anti-B serum – Blood is of group O

5. If clumping occurred with anti-D serum (Colorless), then blood group is Rh +ve

6. If no clumping occurred with anti-D serum, then blood group is Rh-ve

Result: Blood group was determined and found to be ....and Rh ....

Experiment No.: 12

Determination of Erythrocyte Sedimentation Rate (ESR)

Objective:	To determine erythrocyte sedimentation rate (ESR) of my blood
Equipment/ Glassware Required:	1. Disposable syringe and needle. 2. Pasteur pipette with a long thin nozzle. 3. Wintrobe tube and stand –The tube is 12 cm long and closed at its lower end. It is graduated 0 to 10 cm from above downwards from one side (for ESR) and 10 to 0 cm on the other side (for Hct). The Wintrobe's stand can hold up to 3 (or 6) tubes at a time. It is provided with spirit level to ensure that the tubes are held vertical throughout the test.
Chemicals Required:	Sterile swabs moist with 70% alcohol, container with double oxalate mixture or sequestrene.

Principle

In the circulating blood the red cells remain uniformly suspended in the plasma. However, when a sample of blood, to which an anticoagulant has been added, is allowed to stand in a narrow vertical tube i.e. in Wintrobe's haematocrit tube the red cells (sp.gr. =1.095) being heavier (denser) than the colloids plasma (sp.gr.1.032), settle or sediment gradually towards the bottom of the tube. The rate, in mm, at which the red cells sediment in tubes is called ESR, is recorded at the end of one hour.

The settling or sedimentation of red cells in a sample of anticoagulated blood occurs in 3 stages:

1. In the first stage, the RBC's pile up (like a stack of coins), and form rouleaux that become heavier during the first 10-15 minutes.

2. During the second stage, the rouleaux being heavier, sink to the bottom. This stage lasts for 40-45 minutes.

3. In the third stage, there is packing of massed bunches of red cells at the bottom of the blood column. This stage lasts for about 10-12 minutes.

Normal Values

	Normal ESR	Abnormal ESR
Females under 50	0 - 20 mm/hr.	> 20
Males under 50	0 - 15 mm/hr.	> 15
Females over 50	0 - 30 mm/hr.	> 30
Males over 50	0 - 20 mm/hr.	> 20
Children	0 - 10 mm/hr.	> 10

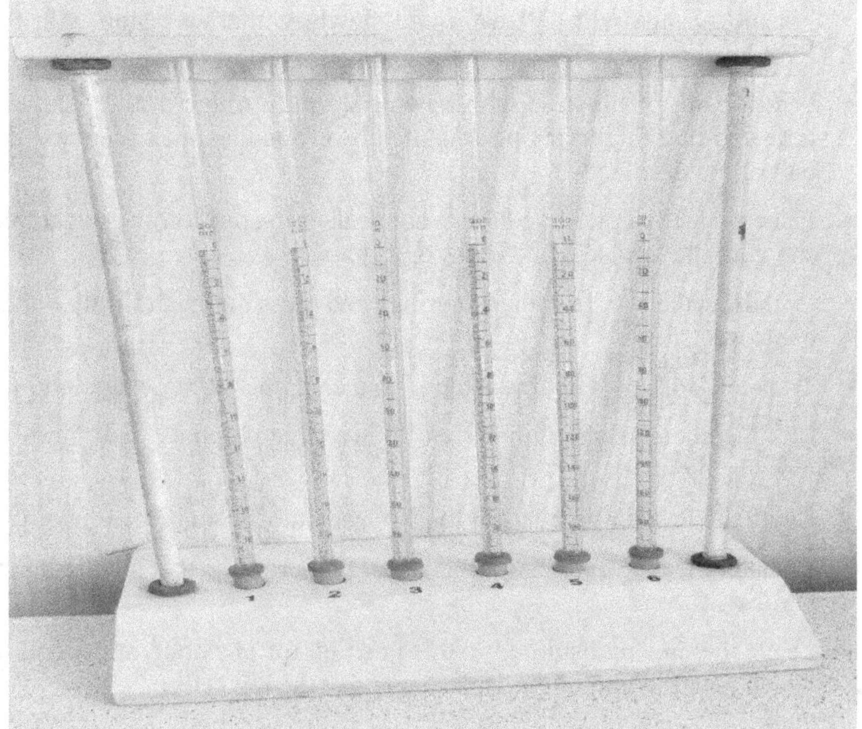

Procedure

Wintrobe's method

- Examine the cubital fossa of his left arm for a "suitable vein".

- Obstruct the venous return either with the armlet of a blood pressure apparatus raising the pressure to 40 mm Hg level or with a strap of broad elastic or by compression of the arm above the vein.

- Clean the skin over the selected vein with spirit and allow it to dry.

- Fix the selected vein by traction on the skin over it with the thumb of your left hand

- Locate a spot on the vein about half a cm below its maximal turgor pressure.

- Puncture at the spot by pushing in the needle firmly and steadily forming an angle of 30° to 50° with the lower arm.

- When the vein is punctured blood enters the syringe and the resistance encountered for pulling the piston is suddenly reduced.

- Fix the syringe with left hand and slowly withdraw piston with the right hand as the blood enters the syringe.

- When 2 mL of blood is withdrawn hold the syringe in the palm the little and ring fingers supporting the piston and the index finger on the butt of the needle.

- Place a piece of sterile cotton wool soaked in spirit on the punctured site with the left hand and press lightly.

- Withdraw the needle with the syringe and press the swab firmly on the punctured site.

- Transfer 2 mL of withdrawn blood to a container of anticoagulant.

- Mix the contents gently but well by inverting the vial a few times or by swirling it.

- Using the Pasteur pipette, fill the wintrobe tube from below upwards.

- Transfer the tube to its stand and adjust the screws so that it will remain vertical.

- Leave the tube undisturbed in this position for one hour, at the end of which read the mm of clear plasma above the red cells.

Caution:

- Do not interchange the tubes provided

- Do not share/exchange syringe and needles

- Do not reuse cotton swab, needle and syringe

- Avoid doing this experiment if you have previous history of bleeding disorder

- Dispose off used cotton swab, needle and syringes only in designated areas or biological waste disposal (yellow) boxes

- Tubes must be kept in upright position to avoid spillages
- Do not shake collection tubes vigorously as it will cause frothing
- Ensure that there are no air bubbles in haematocrit tubes.

Note: *Do not take the reading after ½ hour and then double it to arrive at 1 hour.*

Observation: We studied principle and procedure involved in determination of ESR. The volume of supernatant was read and recorded.

Result: Erythrocyte sedimentation rate (ESR) of my blood is determined to be ....mm/hr.

Experiment No.: 13

Estimation of Hemoglobin

Objective:	To estimate hemoglobin content of blood
Equipment/ Glassware Required:	**A. Sahli's Hemoglobinometer (Hemometer)** 1. **Comparator**: It is rectangular plastic box with a slot in the middle which accommodates the calibrated Hb tube. Non-fading, standardized, golden-brown glass rods are fitted on each side of the slot for matching the color. An opaque white glass or plastic is fitted behind the slot to provide uniform illumination during direct visual color vision. 2. **Hemoglobin tube**: It is calibrated in g Hb % (2-24g %) in yellow color on one side, and in percentage Hb (20-140%) in red color on the other side. There is a brush to clean the tube. 3. **Hemoglobin pipette**: It is a glass capillary pipette with only a single calibration mark of 0.02ml (20 mm^3 or 20 microliters). 4. **Stirrer**: It is a thin glass rod with a flattened end which is used for stirring and mixing the blood and dilute acid. 5. **Ordinary glass dropper** with a rubber teat
Chemicals Required:	**B. Decinormal (N/10) hydrochloric acid solution:** Mixing 36g HCL in distilled water to 1 liter gives Normal HCL; and diluting it 10 times will give N/10 HCL solution. **C. Distill water** **D. Materials for skin prick:** • Sterile lancet/needle • Sterile gauge and cotton swabs • Methylated spirit/ 70% alcohol

Principle

The Hb present in a measured amount of blood is converted by diluted (0.1N) hydrochloric acid into acid hematin, which in dilution is golden brown in color. The intensity of color depends on the concentration of acid hematin which, in turn, depends on the concentration of Hb. The color of the solution, after dilution with water, is matched against golden-brown tinted glass rods by direct vision. The reading is obtained in g%. This method is called as color index method (CIM) or Sahli's Method of Hemoglobin estimation. The normal levels and ranges of Hb at different ages are as follows:

Age	Normal Values
Newborn	18-22 g/dL
At 3 months	14-16 g/dL
3months-1 year	13-15 g/dL
Adult males	13.5-17 g/dL
Adult females	11.5-15.5 g/dL

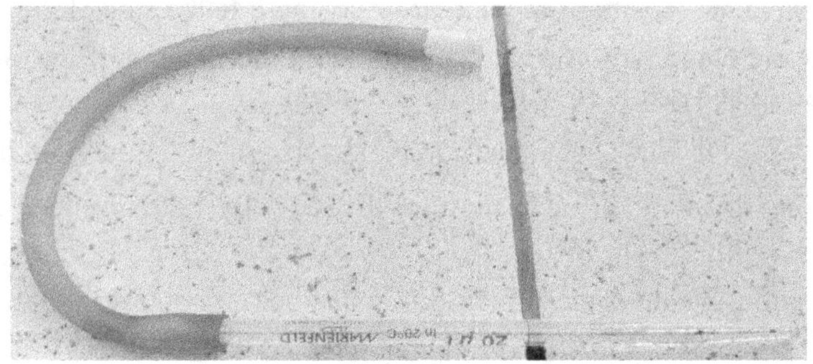

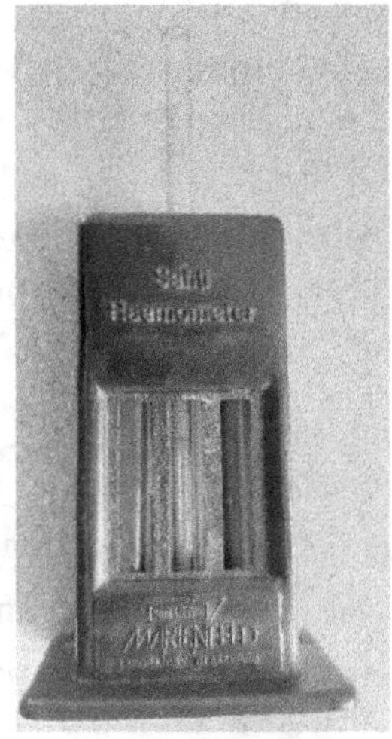

Procedure

- Using a dropper, place 8-10 drops of 0.1N HCL in the HB tube, or up to the mark 20% or 3g, or a little more till the tip of the pipette will submerge, and set it aside.

- Get a finger prick under aseptic conditions; wipe away the first 2 drops of blood. When a large drop of free-flowing blood has formed again, draw blood up to the 20 cm marks (0.02ml). Carefully wipe the blood sticking to the tip of the pipette with a cotton swab, but avoid touching the bore or else blood will be drawn out by capillarity.

- Immediately place the tip of the pipette to the bottom of the acid solution and transfer the blood gently.

- Rinse the Hb pipette with 3-4 times with acid solution.

- Avoid frothing of the mixture.

- Remove the pipette from the tube, touching it to the side of the tube.

- Mix the blood with the acid solution with the flat end of the stirrer by rotating and gently moving it up and down.

- Place the Hb tube back in the comparator and let it stand for 6-8 minutes.

- During this time, the acid ruptures the red cells, releasing their Hb into the solution (hemolysis).

- Duration of time should be 6-8 minutes because shorter duration may leads to incomplete conversion of Hb in to acid hematin whereas longer duration may result in fading of color.

- Diluting and matching the color-
  - Dilute carefully the acid hematin solution with distilled water in drop by drop till its color matches the color of the standard tinted glass rods in the comparator.

- Record the lower meniscus reading of the diluted solution by holding the comparator at eye level, away from your face, against bright but diffused light.

Caution:

- Do not interchange the tubes provided
- Do not share/exchange cotton swab, syringe, needles and lancet
- Do not reuse cotton swab, needle, lancet and syringe
- Avoid doing this experiment if you have previous history of bleeding disorder

- Dispose off used cotton swab, needle, lancet and syringes only in designated areas or biological waste disposal (yellow) boxes

- Tubes must be kept in upright position to avoid spillages

- Do not stir the mixture with sharp end of glass tube vigorously as it will break the tube.

- Ensure that there are no air bubbles in haematocrit tubes.

Observation: I studied the principle and procedure of hemoglobin estimation by taking the average of 3 readings.

	Reading 1	Reading 2	Reading 3	Average
Hb g%				

Reference Range	Your Result	Interpretation
13.5-17 g/dL (Male)		
11.5-15.5g/dL (Female)		

Result: The average of my blood Hb g% was estimated to be.........................

Experiment No.: 14

Determination of Bleeding Time of Blood

Objective:	To determine the bleeding time of my blood by Duke's method.
Equipment/ Glassware Required:	Cotton balls, piece of filter paper, stop watch, sterile blood lancet or needle, sterile cotton/ gauze swabs, 70% alcohol

Principle

The process of stoppage of bleeding after blood vessels are punctured, cut, or otherwise damaged is referred as hemostasis. Hemostasis, which is a homeostatic mechanism to prevent loss of blood, is a result of a complex, natural, physiological response. It involves the following steps.

1. Vasoconstriction (contraction of injured blood vessels)

2. Platelet plug formation

3. Formation of a blood clot

4. Fibrinolysis (dissolution of the clot)

Bleeding time is defined as the time interval between the skin puncture and spontaneous, unassisted (i.e., without pressure) stoppage of bleeding.

Prolonged Bleeding Time is noted in the following conditions:-

a. Low Platelet Count (Thrombocytopenia): Decreased production of platelets and increased destruction of platelets

b. Functional Platelet defects: Due to aspirin, large dose of penicillin, and other drugs, uremia, cirrhosis, leukemia, deficiency of factor VII related antigen.

c. Vessel wall defects: These are genetically acquired but may be inherited.

d. Prolonged treatment with corticosteroids: Also other drugs penicillin, sulphate, and aspirin, etc. may damage vessel walls.

e. Allergic purpura: There is damage to capillary walls by antibodies

f. Infections: Typhus, bacterial endocarditis, hemolytic streptococci

g. Deficiency of vitamin C and connective tissue disorder.

Normal range is 2-7 minutes

Procedure

- Sterilize the finger tip and get a deep finger-prick under aseptic condition to get free- flowing blood.

- Immediately start the stop watch and note the time.

- Absorb/remove the blood drops every 30 seconds by touching the puncture site with the filter paper along its edges, without pressing or squeezing the wound.

- Number the blood spots 1 onwards

- Note the time when bleeding stops, i.e., when there is no trace of blood spot on the filter paper.

- Encircle these spots and number it as well.

- This is the end point.

- Count the number of blood spots and express your results in minutes and seconds.

Caution:

- Do not keep the filter paper on the table and then press your wound on it.

- Record the time of puncturing and application to fingertip

- Do not share/exchange cotton swab, filter paper, needles and lancet

- Do not reuse cotton swab, needle, lancet and syringe

- Avoid doing this experiment if you have previous history of bleeding disorder

- Dispose off used cotton swab, needle, lancet and filter papers only in designated areas or biological waste disposal (yellow) boxes

Normal bleeding time: 2-7 minutes

Observation: The principle, procedure in bleeding time are studied and practiced.

Reference Range	Your Result	Interpretation
2-7 minutes (Bleeding Time)		

Result: The bleeding time of my blood was calculated to be
……………………….. .

Experiment No.: 15

Determination of Clotting Time of Blood

Objective:	To determine the clotting time of blood.
Equipment/ Glassware Required:	Cotton balls, capillary glass tube, stop watch, sterile blood lancet or needle, sterile cotton/ gauze swabs, 70% alcohol

Principle: Normally blood remains in liquid form in blood vessels, but when drawn from the body it changes into semisolid gel. The clotting time is defined as the time taken to coagulate (gel) the blood after rupture of blood vessel. It is also an interval between the entry of blood into the glass capillary, or a syringe, and formation of fibrin threads.

Clotting time is increased in the following conditions:

- *Hereditary coagulation disorder*
  I.   Due to hemophiliac- A, B, C, D.
  II. Afibrinogenemia and dysfibrinogenemia- The concentration of fibrinogen may be greatly reduced or absent or it may be chemically abnormal.

- *Acquired coagulation disorders*- These develop in a variety of disease such as:
  I.   Vitamin K deficiency – Since vitamin K act as a cofactor in the synthesis of prothrombin, and factors VII, IX and X.
  II. Liver diseases- This causes decrease in all clotting factors except VII, reduced uptake of vitamin K, and abnormalities of platelet function.
  III. Intravascular clotting- Clotting factors are used up and bleeding may occur.
  IV. Anticoagulant therapy- Patients receiving heparin or warfarin.

Clotting time is decreased in the physiological conditions –Malnutrition, parturition.

Normal range is 3-6 minutes

Procedure

- Sterilize the fingertip and take a bold prick to have free flow of blood.

- Absorb the first 2 drops of blood on a separate filter paper and allow a large drop to form.

- Now dip one end of the capillary tube in the blood; the blood rises into the tube by capillary action. This can be enhanced by keeping its open end at a lower level.

- Note the time when blood starts to enter the tube.

- This is the zero time.

- Hold the capillary tube between the palms of your hands to keep the blood near body temperature.

- Gently break off 1 cm bits of glass tube from one end at intervals of 30 seconds, and look for the formation of fibrin threads between the broken ends.

- The end-point is reached when fibrin threads span a gap of 5 mm between the broken ends (rope formation).

- Note the time.

Normal clotting time =3-6 minutes

Caution:

- Do not press glass capillaries in to your wound

- Record the time of entry of blood in glass capillary tube

- Do not share/exchange cotton swab, glass capillary, needles and lancet

- Do not reuse cotton swab, needle, lancet and syringe

- Avoid doing this experiment if you have previous history of bleeding disorder

- Dispose off used cotton swab, needle, lancet, glass capillary and filter papers only in designated areas or biological waste disposal (yellow) boxes

Observation: The principle, procedure in blood clotting are studied and practiced.

Reference Range	Your Result	Interpretation
3-6 minutes (Clotting Time)		

Result: The clotting time of my blood was calculated to be ……………………………..

Experiment No.: 16

White Blood Cell (WBC) Count

Objective:	To determine white blood cell (WBC) counts of the blood
Equipment / Glassware Required:	WBC pipette, Improved Neubauer chamber, cover slip, compound microscope, disposable blood lancet/ pricking needle, sterile cotton/gauze swabs, 70% alcohol.
Chemicals Required:	Turk's fluid Composition is Glacial acetic acid = 1.5ml (hemolyzes RBCs without affecting WBCs), Gentian violet (1% solution) =1.5ml (it stains the nuclei of leucocytes) and distilled water to 100ml.

Principle

WBCs or leucocytes constitute the major defense system of the body against invasion by bacteria, viruses, fungi, toxins and other foreign invaders. Their number increases or decreases in many diseases. The normal count in adults ranges between 4000-11000/mm^3. The count after birth may be as high as 18000 to 20000/mm^3, the normal levels being reached in a few years. Leucocytosis is the increase in number of WBCs beyond 11000/mm^3. Leucopenia is the decrease in the number of WBCs below the normal level.

A sample of blood is diluted with a diluting fluid which destroys the red cells and stains the nuclei of the leucocytes and also brought the number of WBC to a level which could be counted easily. The cells are then counted in a counting chamber and their number in undiluted blood reported as leucocytes/cmm. This method is also called as total leucocyte count (TLC).

Normal Count

Age range	WBC count (per cmm of blood)
Newborns	9,000 to 30,000
Children under 2	6,200 to 17,000
Children over 2 and adults	5,000 to 10,000

Neubauer Chamber

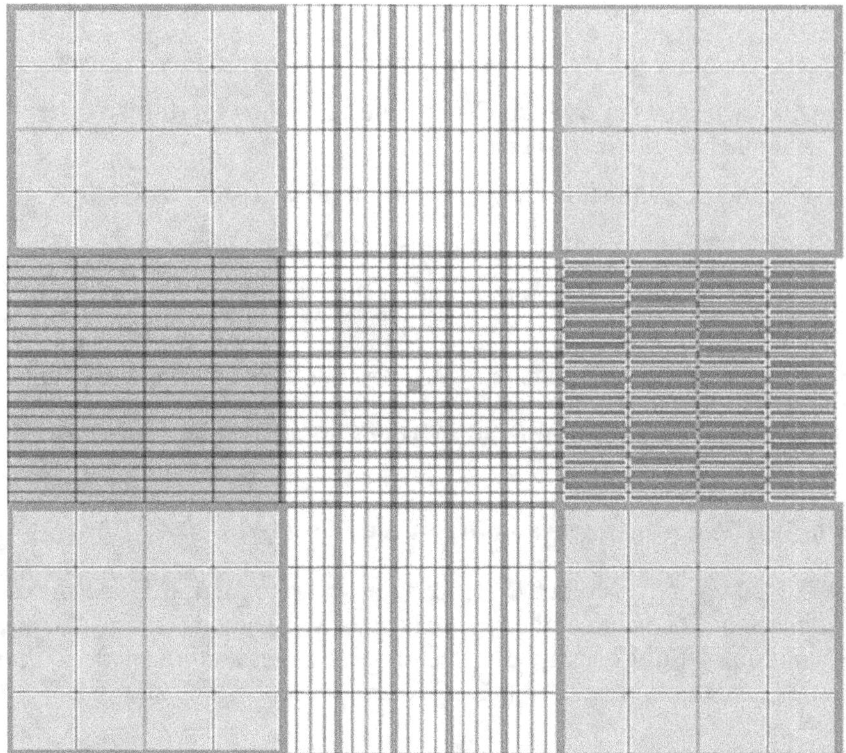

Procedure

- Rinse the WBC pipette (with white head and white bead) and set aside.

- Take 1 ml of Turk's fluid in a watch glass.

- Place the counting chamber on the microscope stage.

- Adjust the illumination, and focus the right upper group of 16 WBC squares. You will see all the squares in one field.

- Observe all the aseptic precautions, get a finger-prick, discard the first 2 drops of blood, and let a good-sized drop to form.

- Filling the pipette- Dip the tip of the pipette in the edge of the drop, draw blood to the mark 0.5 and suck Turk's fluid to the mark 11.

- Mix the contents of the bulb thoroughly for 3-4 minutes.

- Charging the chamber- Discard the first 2 drops of fluid from the pipette and charge the chamber.

- The chamber should neither be over-charged nor under-charged.

- Allow the cells to settle for 3-4 minutes, and then carefully transfer the chamber to the microscope.

- Use the fine adjustment again and try to identify the WBCs.

- Switch to high magnification and study the leucocytes.

- Count the cells in the 4 groups of 16 squares each, i.e., in a total of 64 squares.

- Draw appropriate squares in your workbook for entering the counts.

Total WBC count = number of cells counted x Total area counted x Dilution factor

Total WBC count/cmm = number of cells counted x 10/4 × 20

NOTE: In leucocytes pipette, blood is drawn up to mark 0.5, and filled in up to mark 11. The bulb of the pipette is made such that it contains 10 times the volume of fluid contained in the stem of pipette up to mark 1. So if blood is taken up to mark 0.5 (i.e. ½), then dilution will be 20 times.

Caution

- Sterilize your fingertip properly

- Use only sterilized needle or lancet

- Do not share/exchange cotton swab, needles and lancet

- Do not reuse cotton swab, needle, lancet and syringe

- Avoid doing this experiment if you have previous history of bleeding disorder

- Dispose-off used cotton swab, needle, lancet, and filter papers only in designated areas or biological waste disposal (yellow) boxes

- Wash the WBC pipette as soon as possible to avoid blood clotting in the pipette.

- Wash Neubauer chamber properly before you return

- Cover the counting area of the chamber with cover slip before you observe it in microscope.

Observation:

These WBCs are round in shapes, the clear unstained cytoplasm, and the deep blue-violet nuclei which appear lobed in some cells and single in others. Few remnants the red cell membranes called ghost cells are also faintly visible.

Reference Range	Your Result	Interpretation
5,000 to 10,000 per cmm of blood		

Result: The principle and procedure in white blood cell count was learned and practiced using improved Neubauer chamber. White blood cell (WBC) count of my blood was calculated to be…………………………..

Experiment No.: 17

Determination of RBC Count

Objective:	Estimation of total red blood corpuscles (RBC) count
Equipment/ Glassware Required:	RBC Pipette, Improved Neubauer chamber, cover slip, compound microscope, disposable blood lancet/ pricking needle,70% alcohol, sterile cotton swabs.
Chemicals Required:	Hayem's fluid (RBC diluting fluid)- Composition - Sodium chloride- 0.5g, Sodium sulphate-2.5g, Mercuric chloride-0.25g, Distilled water- 100ml

Principle

The RBCs are non-nucleated cells with a life span of 120 days and are formed by erythropoiesis. The normal RBC count ranges from 4.75-6.0 million/mm^3 in males, and 4.0-5.5 million mm^3. The blood is diluted 200 times in a red cell pipette and the cells are counted in the counting chamber. Knowing the dilution employed, their number in undiluted blood can be calculated. RBCs are blood cells that contain HB and carry oxygen. The RBC count provides valuable information in diagnosing the type of anemia in Patients.

Anemia is a condition in which the oxygen carrying capacity of blood is reduced. It is due to types decreased concentration of Hb, usually below 11-12g/dl as a result of decrease in RBCs below 4-4.5 million/mm^3. Types of anemia are Iron deficiency anemia, hemorrhagic anemia, Hemolytic anemia-inherited and acquired (drug, parasite), pernicious anemia, aplastic anemia, anemia due to chronic disease. *Polycythemia*- It refers to increase in the number of red cells above the normal level.

Normal RBC range

Men	4.7-6.1 million cells per microliter
Women	4.2-5.4 million cells per microliter
Children	4.0 – 5.5 million cells per microliter

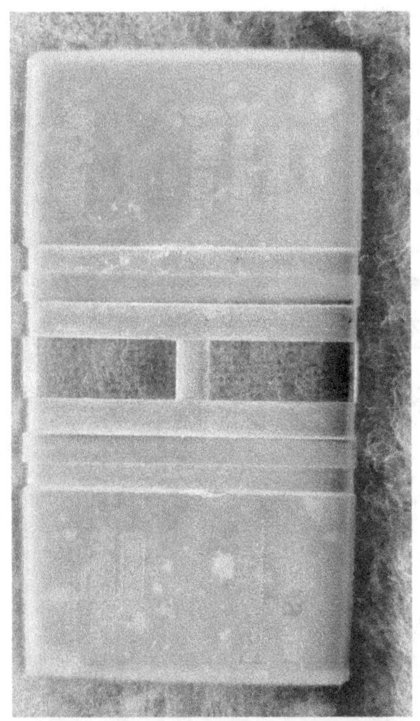

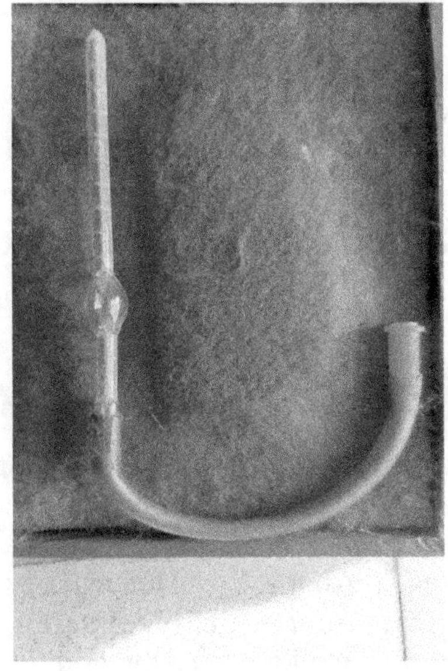

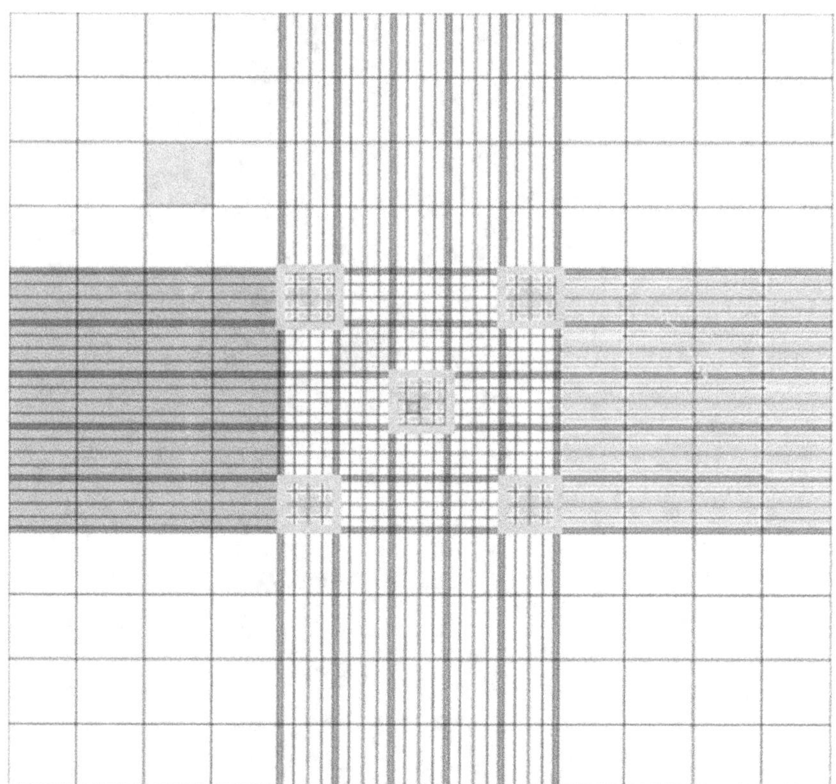

RBC/cmm = number of cell counted x dilution factor x depth x area counted

RBC/cmm = ... x 200 x 10 x 5

Procedure

- Place about 2ml of Hayem's fluid in a watch glass.

- Examine the chamber, with the coverslip centred on it, under low magnification. Adjust the illumination and focus the central 1mm square (RBC square on the counting grid) containing 25 groups of 16 smallest squares each. All these squares will be visible in one field. Do not change the focus or the field. Admitting too much light is a common cause of the inability to see the grid lines and squares clearly.

- Move the chamber to your work-table for charging it with diluted blood.

- Filling the pipette with blood and diluting it. - Get a finger-prick. Wipe the first 2 drops of blood and fill the pipette from a fresh drop of blood up to the mark 0.5. Suck Hayem's fluid to the mark 101 and mix the contents of the bulb for 3-4 minutes.

- Charging the chamber- Observing all the precautions, fill the chamber with diluted blood. Since the RBC pipette is a slow speed pipette, it will need to be kept at an angle of 70-80-degree while charging the chamber.

- Move the chamber to the microscope and focus the grid once again to see the central 1mm square with the red cells distributed all over.

- Wait for 3-4minutes for the cells to settle down because they cannot be counted when they are moving and changing their positions due to currents in the fluid. During this time draw 5 groups of 16 squares each, showing their relative positions.

- Counting the cells – Switch over to high magnification and check the distribution of cells, if they are unevenly distributed, i.e., bunched at some places and scanty at others, the chamber has to be washed, dried, and recharged.

- Move the chamber carefully and bring the left upper corner block of 16 smallest squares in the field of view. Thus counting will have been done in 80 smallest squares, i.e., in 5 blocks of 16 squares each.

- Add up the number of cells in each of the 5 blocks of 16 smallest squares. A difference of more than 20 between any 2 blocks indicates uneven distribution.

❖ **Rules for counting**

1. Cells lying on the tramp or triple lines do not form part of the boundary of that square.

2. Cells lying within a square are to be counted with that square.

3. Cells lying on or touching its upper horizontal and left vertical lines are to be counted with that particular square.

4. Cells lying on or touching its lower horizontal and right vertical lines are to be omitted from that square because they will be counted with the adjacent squares

Note: In erythrocytes pipette blood is drawn upto 0.5 and filled upto mark 101. The bulb of the pipette is made such that is contains 100 times the volume of fluid contained in the stem of the pipette upto the mark. So if blood is taken up to mark1, then dilution is 1:100. If blood is taken upto mark 0.5 (i.e. ½), then dilution will be 1:200.

Observation: The microscopic structure of RBC, principles and procedure involved in RBC determination were learned and practiced.

Reference Range	Your Result	Interpretation
4.7-6.1 million cells per microliter		
4.2-5.4 million cells per microliter		

Result: Total red blood corpuscles (RBC) count of blood was found to be ……………………..

Experiment No.: 18

Differential Count of the Blood

Objective:	To study the differential count of the blood sample.
Equipment/ Glassware Required:	Glass slide, spreader slide, microscope,
Chemicals Required:	Eosin (red) and methylene blue dyes

Principle

The differential blood count gives the relative percentage of each type of white blood cells (WBCs) and also helps to reveal abnormal white blood cell populations (for example, blasts, immature granulocytes, and circulating lymphoma cells in the peripheral blood).

DIFFERENTIAL WHITE BLOOD CELLS NORMAL COUNT

CELL TYPE	NORMAL VALUE (%)	ELEVATED LEVELS MAY INDICATE
NEUTROPHILS	54-62	Bacterial infections, stress
LYMPHOCYTE	25-33	Mononucleosis, whooping cough, viral infections
MONOCYTE	3-9	Malaria, tuberculosis, fungal infections
EOSINOPHILS	1-3	Allergic reactions, autoimmune disease, parasitic worms
BASOPHILS	<1	Cancer, chicken pox, hypothyroidism

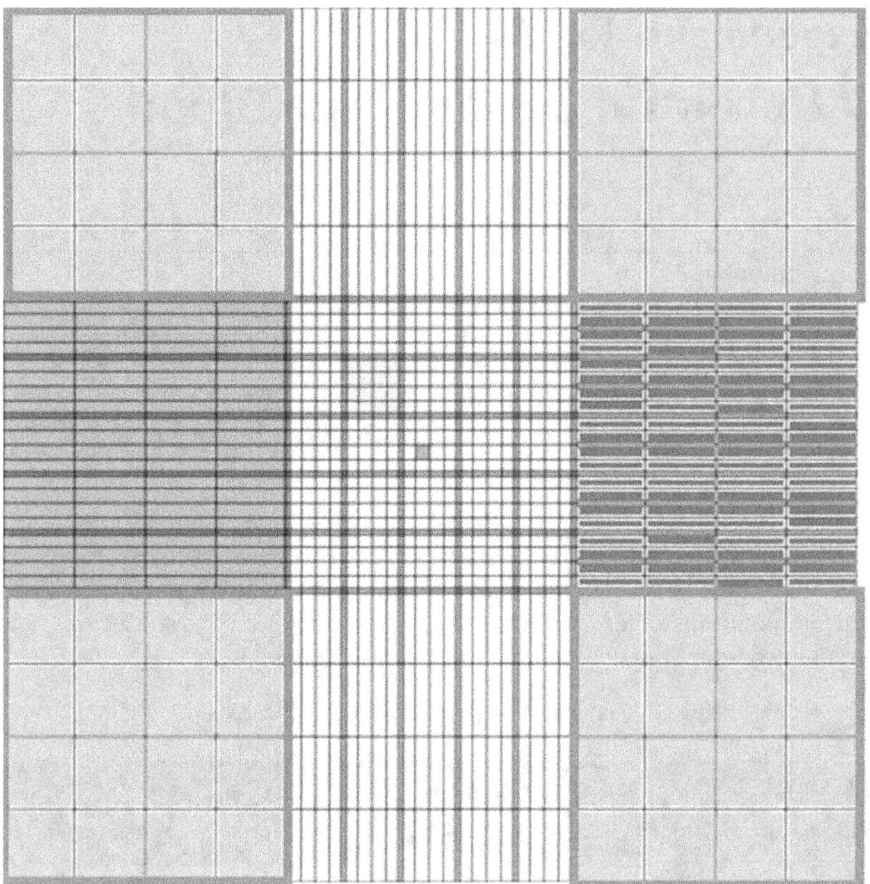

Procedure

- Take a glass slide and put a drop of blood at the one end of it.

- Using a spreader glass slide, make a film keeping the spreader slide at the angle of 30^0-40^0.

- Stain the film after drying with mixture of eosin (red) and methylene blue dyes.

- Confirm that the film is good and well stained.

- Mount & focus the oil immersion lens accurately.

- Bring the left upper corner, of the film in view.

- Identify all the cells seen.

- Draw columns and label them for each type of the cells.

- Denote each cell by an inclined line fifth line crossing the group of four in the appropriate column.

- Do not leave any cell unidentified or unentered.

- Move the slide towards the left along the same horizontal axis to bring the adjacent field in view. (Visual field moves towards right.). Identify every cell and enter the observations till you reach the right upper corner of the film.

- Now shift the slide up, to bring the lower adjacent field comes in view (The visual field moves down). Identify and enter your observations. Go on counting by moving the slide to the right till the left end comes under the objective. Then shift lower down again and go on counting towards the right again and so on.

Observation

The students should count the number of cells and convert the count into percentage and then compare with the given table:

Reference Range		Your Result	Interpretation
Neutrophils	54-62		
Lymphocytes	25-33		
Monocytes	3-9		
Eosinophils	1-3		
Basophils	<1		

Result: The differential features of Neutrophil, Eosinophil, Basophil, Lymphocyte and Monocyte were studied and counted to be …………………………………………….. and …………….. respectively.

Experiment No: 19

Neurological Examination

Objective:	To study and practice the techniques of neurological examination
Equipment/ Glassware Required:	Chart/model/specimen of human cranial nerves

Principle

Any slight irregularity found during a comprehensive neurologic examination might be a sign of a neurological injury. Early referral to a neurologist or treatment can save more harm from occurring. A comprehensive neurologic evaluation will look at ones mental state, the cranial nerves, the motor and sensory function, the reflexes, the cerebellum, and other vital signs. The evaluation of cranial nerves, will be the focus of this experiment. Despite the fact that this isn't a thorough neurologic examination, it will provide important clinical signal.

Procedure

Examination of Cranial Nerves

Cranial nerve I (olfactory): It is a test to gauge one's sense of smell. Ask your friend to close his/her eyes and identify at least two familiar smells of items such as coffee, lemon, or orange. If your friend is unable to identify the object, this can indicate neurological damage.

Cranial nerve (optic): The Rosenbaum near-vision card and Snellen chart are used in this visual acuity test. Hold the chart at a distance of 14 inches. Use a wall clock or a white board to read similar-sized letters if the chart is not accessible. If unable to read, a neurological disability may be present.

Cranial nerve III (oculomotor): This examination is used to measure the corneal light reflex. To test the eye's motor function, ask your friend to move their eyes up, down, side to side, and diagonally. You might even request that your friend follow the penlight's light in different directions.

Examine the pupils' dimensions, symmetry, and responses to light in the papillaries as well.

Opioid overdose is frequently present if the pupils are not responding and are pinpoint. Sedatives and opioids can also cause sluggish (slowly constricting) pupils. A fixed and dilated pupil is often a very alarming and late indication of neurological impairment.

Cranial nerve IV (trochlear nerve): This nerve also helps with the movement of the eyes. Above test may be helpful in deriving inference.

Cranial nerve V (trigeminal): Ask your friend to close his eyes, then touch him with a wisp of cotton on each side of his forehead, face, and jaw to evaluate the sensory function of the trigeminal nerve. Next, apply the safety pin's point to the same three spots to assess their pain threshold. Request that he differentiate and describe the two feelings. Test the patient's capacity to distinguish between warm and cold as well. For the cold test, you may place a few ice cubes in a glove, and for the heated test, you can use a heel warmer. Ask him to bite his teeth as you feel the masseter and temporal muscles to evaluate the motor component. The muscular contraction should be equally strong on both sides. Test your friend's corneal reaction if he isn't paying attention by gently stroking the cornea with a tiny piece of cotton. Watch for the eyes to blink normally as a response. (Note: Individuals who are awake are not tested for corneal reflexes.) The capacity to feel the face, the interior of the mouth, and to move the muscles used for chewing are just a few of the many functions that are made possible by this nerve.

Cranial nerve VI (abducens nerve): This nerve helps with the movement of the eyes. The patient may be asked to follow a light or finger to move the eyes.

Cranial nerve VII (facial nerve): This nerve controls a number of processes, including taste and facial muscle movement. The patient could be asked to name several flavours (sweet, sour, and bitter), or they might be instructed to smile, move their cheeks, or expose their teeth. You are seeking symmetry over the entire face.

Cranial nerve VIII (acoustic nerve): The hearing nerve is located here. The individual could get a hearing test. To find out if your friend can hear the sound, rub your fingers together next to each ear. Perform the Romberg test since this nerve is involved in balance as well. To do this test, ask the person to remain still for 30 seconds with their eyes open, then for 30 seconds with their eyes closed. If they become unsteady, this is a positive Romberg test and may indicate that the acoustic nerve is not operating at its best.

Cranial nerve IX (glossopharyngeal nerve): Taste and swallowing are both controlled by this nerve. Once more, you may ask your friend to name the various flavours on their tongue's back. One may examine the gag reflex. Pay attention to the voice. Then, instruct the patient to open wide and utter "ah" as you press the tip of a tongue blade on the back of his or her throat. Keep an eye out for the uvula's midline location, as well as symmetrical upward migration of the soft palate and uvula.

Cranial nerve X (vagus nerve): The gag reflex, the capacity to swallow, some taste, and a portion of speech are all primarily controlled by this nerve. A tongue blade may be used to trigger the gag reflex after the patient is requested to swallow.

Cranial nerve X (vagus nerve): The pharynx serves primarily as a motor function test for the vagus nerve, which is simultaneously sensory and motor. Asking your friend to talk and swallow can help you evaluate how it works. Hoarseness is a symptom of nerve damage.

Cranial nerve XI (accessory nerve): The trapezius and sternocleidomastoid are both innervated by the accessory nerve. The neck and shoulders are moved by means of this nerve. Ask your friend to raise their shoulders by putting your hands on their shoulders. Equal power should be applied to both shoulders as they rise. Place a palm against one cheek and ask the subject to turn their head against resistance to test the sternoclei domastroid. Do the same with the other cheek. This is the muscular strength test.

Cranial nerve XII (hypoglossal nerve). The mobility of the tongue is mostly controlled by the last cranial nerve. Your friend can be told to talk while sticking out his or her tongue. Check the symmetry of your friend's tongue. Without any tremors or muscular twitches, the tongue should be in the middle. The tongue might deviate to one side, which indicates neurological damage.

Observation: We learned the theory and skill involved in neurological examination with the help of my friend.

Result: Neurological examination of my friend shows that there is no neurological deficit/ a neurological deficit in cranial nerves
....

Experiment No.: 20

Measurement of Blood Pressure

Objective:	To measure the blood pressure using BP apparatus
Equipment:	Stethoscope, Sphygmomanometer, digital BP apparatus

Principle

Blood pressure refers to the force exerted by the blood as it presses against and attempts to stretch the walls of blood vessels. It is an important clinical procedure as it provides valuable information about the cardiovascular system under normal and disease conditions.

A sufficient length of a single artery is selected in the arm (brachial artery). The artery is first compressed by inflating a rubber bag (connected to the manometer) placed around the arm (or thigh) to stop the blood flow through the occluded section of the artery. The pressure is then released slowly and the flow of blood through the obstructed segment of the artery is studied by:

1. Feeling the pulse- The palpatory method.

2. Observing the oscillations of the mercury column-The oscillometric method, and

3. Listening to the sounds produced in the part of the artery just below the obstructed segment- the auscultatory method.

Stethoscope: The instrument has the following 3 parts:

i. *The chest-piece-* The chest-piece has two end pieces-a bell and a flat diaphragm.

ii. *The rubber tubing-* It is a single soft-rubber pressure tube (3mm diameter) leads from the chest-piece to a metal Y-shaped connector.

iii. *The ear-frame-*It consists of two curved metallic tubes joined together with a flat U-shaped spring which keeps them pulled together. The upper ends of the tubes are curved so that they correspond to the curve of the external auditory meatus. Two plastic knobs threaded over the ends of the tubes fit snugly in the ear.

Sphygmomanometer: It is an instrument routinely used for recording arterial blood pressure. It consists of the following parts:

a) *Mercury manometer*: The manometer is fitted in the lid of the instrument. One arm of the manometer is the reservoir for mercury- a broad and short well that contains enough mercury to be driven up in the other limb- the graduated glass tube.

b) *Graduated tube*: The manometer glass tube is graduated in mm from 0 to 300, each division representing 2 mm, though actually slightly less than 2 mm.

A stopcock between the two limbs, when closed, prevents the mercury from entering the glass tube. The one-way valve fitted at the top of the mercury well prevents spilling of mercury when the lid is closed, while allowing pressure to be transmitted from the rubber bag to the mercury reservoir. A spring-loaded clip at the top of the tube keeps it firmly pressed into a rubber washer at its lower end to prevent leakage of mercury.

c) *The armlet* (rubber bag; Riva Rocci cuff): The cuff as it is usually called, consist of an inflatable rubber bag, 24cm x 12cm, which is fitted with 2 rubber tubes- one connecting it to the mercury reservoir and the other to a rubber bulb (air pump). The bag is enclosed in a long strip of inelastic cloth with a long tapering free end. The cloth covering keeps the rubber bag in position around the arm when pressure is being measured. The recommended width of the bag in different age groups is as under:

Infants (below 1 year): 2.5 cm

Below 4 years: 5 cm

Below 8 years: 8 cm

Adults   : 12 cm

d) *Air pump (rubber bulb)*: It is an oval-shaped rubber bulb of a size that conveniently fits into one's fist. It has a one-way valve at its free end, and a leak-valve with a knurled screw, at the other where the rubber tube leading to the cuff is attached. The cuff can be inflated by turning the leak valve screw clockwise, and alternately compressing and releasing the bulb. Deflation of the bag is achieved by turning this screw anticlockwise.

Normal Range

Age	Male		Female	
	SBP	DBP	SBP	DBP
21-25	120.5	78.5	115.5	70.5
26-30	119.5	76.5	113.5	71.5
31-35	114.5	75.5	110.5	72.5
36-40	120.5	75.5	112.5	74.5
41-45	115.5	78.5	116.5	73.5
46-50	119.5	80.5	124	78.5
51-55	125.5	80.5	122.55	74.5
56-60	129.5	79.5	132.5	78.5
61-65	143.5	76.5	130.5	77.5

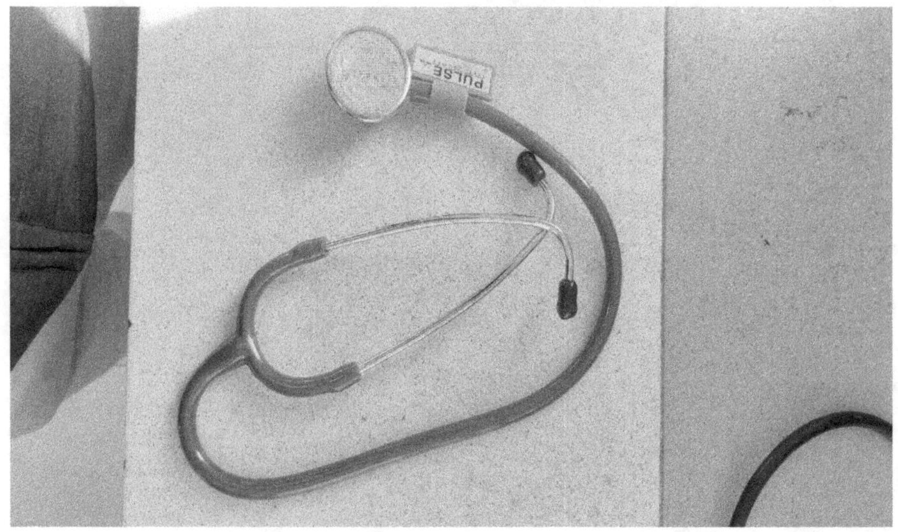

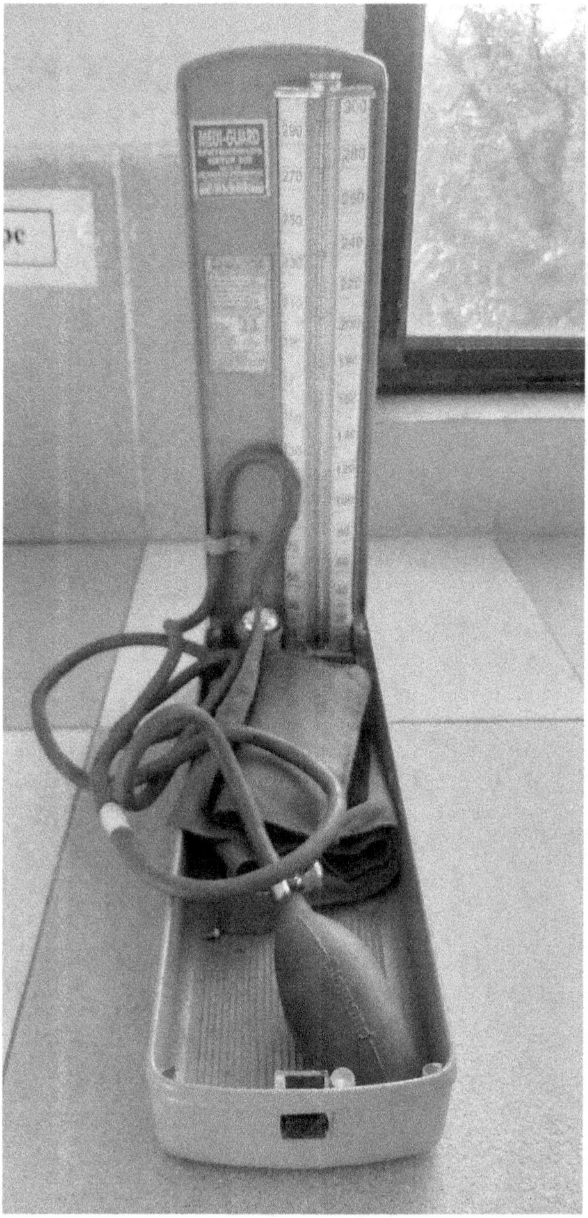

Procedure

Auscultatory method:

1. Calm down the subject and ask them to lie down or sit in relaxed condition.

2. Place the cuff over the upper arm at the level of heart.

3. Locate the brachial artery. Mark the point of arterial pulsation with a sketch pen.

4. Place the chest-piece of the stethoscope on this point and keep it in position with your fingers and the thumb of the left hand (if you are right-handed).

5. Inflate the cuff rapidly, by compressing and releasing the air pump alternately. Raise the pressure to about 140 mm Hg.

6. Lower the pressure gradually until a clear, sharp, tapping sound is heard. Continue to lower the pressure and try to note a change in the character of the sounds.

7. Note the reading at muffling and another at disappearance of sounds, after which deflate the cuff quickly.

8. Take 3 readings with the auscultatory method of right arm.

Observation: The principle and procedure involved in regulation of blood pressure was learned and measured blood pressure of my friend.

Body Posture	Digital BP Apparatus		Mercury Manometer	
	SBP	DBP	SBP	DBP
Sitting (Left Arm)				
Sitting (Right Arm)				
Standing (Left Arm)				
Standing (Right Arm)				
Supine (Left Arm)				
Supine (Right Arm)				
After walking for 5 minutes (Left Arm)				
After walking for 5 minutes (Right Arm)				

Result: The average blood pressure of my friend is found to be
....

Experiment No.: 21

Recording Body Temperature

Objective:	To record the body temperature using mercury, digital and IR thermometer.
Equipment/ Glassware Required:	Thermometers (mercury, digital and IR)

Principle

The measurement of the body temperature is very common and important clinical investigation. Altered body temperature signifies disease condition. Elevated body temperature is called as fever and usually accompany with disease condition. The body temperature differs from one body site to other, organ to organ, through age, through time of the day, environment etc.

The body temperature is measured using thermometer. Various types of thermometers are present today, to measure the body temperature. These includes, mercury thermometer, digital thermometer, and IR thermometer.

The mercury thermometer works by the expansion of mercury filled inside the tube aligned with the scale. The digital thermometer contains sensors like thermocouples, resistance temperature detectors (RTD) which sense the change in temperature and reflect that as numerical display. The IR thermometers work using IR detectors which convert the radiant energy into electrical energy.

Average normal body temperature by age

Age	Oral	Rectal/Ear	Armpit
0–12 months	95.8–99.3°F (36.7–37.3°C)	96.8–100.3°F (37–37.9°C)	94.8–98.3°F (36.4–37.3°C)

Table *contd...*

Age	Oral	Rectal/Ear	Armpit
Children	97.6–99.3°F (36.4–37.4°C)	98.6–100.3°F (37–37.9°C)	96.6–98.3°F (35.9–36.83°C)
Adults	96–98°F (35.6–36.7°C)	97–99°F (36.1–37.2°C)	95–97°F (35–36.1°C)
Adults over age 65	93–98.6°F (33.9–37°C)	94–99.6°F (34.4–37.6°C)	92–97.6°F (33.3–36.4°C)

Severity of Fever

Temperature	Inference
at least 100.4°F (38°C)	Fever
above 103.1°F (39.5°C)	high fever
above 105.8°F (41°C)	very high fever

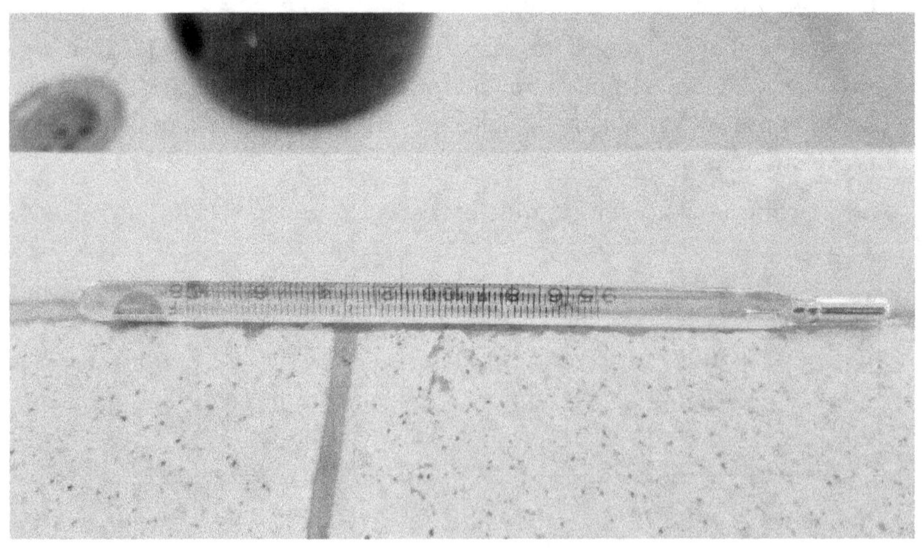

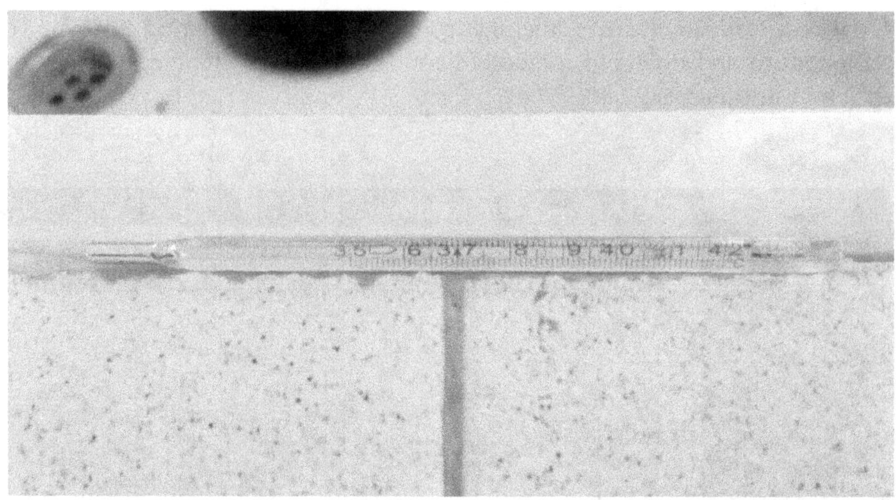

Procedure

Mercury thermometer:

1. Take out the thermometer carefully and look for the mercury level in the scale.

2. Put the bulb of thermometer either below the tongue or under your armpit.

3. Wait for sometime and then look for the increased level of mercury in the tube, that's the temperature of the body.

4. Clean the bulb with alcohol before storing the thermometer again.

Digital thermometer:

1. Take the digital thermometer and switch it on.

2. When screen becomes active, place the thermometer either below the tongue or under the armpit.

3. Wait till the thermometer beeps, after the beep take it out and look for the temperature reading.

4. Clean the bulb with alcohol before storing.

IR thermometer:

1. Take the thermometer and switch it on.

2. When screen becomes active, point the instrument towards the back of wrist or head of the subject and look for the reading.

Observation: We learned the theory involved in regulating core body temperature and different methods of measuring body temperature using different instruments.

Body Temperature	Reference Range	Your Result		
		Digital Thermometer	Merury Thermometer	IR Thermometer
Oral	96–98°F (35.6–36.7°C)			
Ear	97–99°F (36.1–37.2°C)			
Armpit	95–97°F (35–36.1°C)			

Result: My body temperature using mercury thermometer, digital thermometer and IR thermometer were measured to be …………………….., …………….. and ………………… respectively.

Experiment No.: 22

Determination of Pulse/Heart Rate

Objective:	To determine the pulse/heart rate.
Equipment/ Glassware Required:	Stopwatch

Principle

The pulse rate is a measurement of the heart rate, or the number of times the heart beats per minute. As the heart pushes blood through the arteries, the arteries expand and contract with the flow of the blood. Taking a pulse not only measures the heart rate, but also can indicate the heart rhythm and strength of the pulse.

The normal pulse for healthy adults ranges from 60 to 100 beats per minute. The pulse rate may fluctuate and increase with exercise, illness, injury, and emotions.

The pulse rate varies with age. The pulse rate of fetus is about 140 per minute. In a newly born infant it is about 130/minute. At the age of five it is reduced to about 90/minute. At the age of 10 years to 80, at the age of 15 years to 75/minute, and at the age of 20 it comes to about 70 per minute. It remains constant throughout the life after this age. Slow pulse rate is called bradycardia and high pulse rate is called tachycardia.

Sites for Pulse Examination: Radial, ulner, dorsalis pedis and the temporal vessels are the usual sites. All the sites should be examined in the same manner. Abnormalities detected at only one site are likely to be helpful in localization of the disease.

Pulse rate by age		Interpretation	
		Pulse	**Possible cause**
Neonate (<28 days)	100-205		
Infant (1 month – 1 year)	100-190	Rapid, regular and full	Exertion, fear, fever, hypertension
Toddler (1-2 years)	98-140	Rapid, regular and weak	Hypovolaemic shock
Pre-school (2-5 years)	80-120	Slow	Head injury, drug use, poisons, cardiac problems
6-11 years	75-118	Irregular	This is quite common and not necessarily a problem.
12 years - adult	60-100		
Athlete	40-60		

Procedure

- As the heart forces blood through the arteries, the beats can be felt by firmly pressing on the arteries, which are located close to the surface of the skin at certain points of the body like wrist.

- Using the first and second finger tips, press firmly but gently on the arteries until you feel a pulse.

- Begin counting the pulse.

- Count your pulse for 60 seconds and record the number.

Observation: We learned the theory involved in regulating heart rate/ pulse rate and measured pulse rate at Radial, Ulner, Dorsalis pedis and the Temporal vessels sites of body.

Reference Range		Your Result	Interpretation
12 years - adult	60-100		
	Radian		
	Ulnar		
	Dorsalis pedis		
	Temporal vessel		

Result: The pulse rate measured at Radial, Ulner, Dorsalis pedis and the Temporal vessels sites of body was found to be ……………, ………………..., ………………., and ……………... respectively.

Experiment No.: 23

Determination of Respiratory Rate

Objective:	To determine the respiratory rate
Equipment/ Glassware Required:	Stopwatch

Principle

Respiratory rate is one of the most vital function of the body and is defined as the number of breaths per minute. The respiratory rate determines the functional efficiency of lungs and any further respiratory disorder. For humans, the typical respiratory rate for a healthy adult at rest is 12–16 breaths per minute. The change in pattern and rate of respiration is a reflection of change in body's physiology and delivery of oxygen to vital organs and tissues.

Respiration rate is well controlled and regulated by nervous, muscular, hormonal and other systems. Lower rate of respiration is a reflection of CNS depression and higher rate of respiration indicates other abnormality. Furthermore,

Age	Normal range
birth to 6 weeks	30–40 breaths per minute
6 months	25–40 breaths per minute
3 years	20–30 breaths per minute
6 years	18–25 breaths per minute
10 years	17–23 breaths per minute
Adults	15–18 breaths per minute
Elderly $\geq$ 65 years old	12–28 breaths per minute
Elderly $\geq$ 80 years old	10-30 breaths per minute

Procedure

- Sit down and try to relax.

- It's best to take your respiratory rate while sitting up in a chair or in bed.
- Measure your breathing rate by counting the number of times your chest or abdomen rises over the course of one minute.
- Start stopwatch
- Count number of breaths for 1 minute
- Stop stopwatch
- Record this number.

Observation: We learned the theory involved in regulating respiration at different body postures.

Body posture and activities	Your results	Interpretation
Sitting		
Standing		
After 50 steps		
Supine		
After skipping		

Result: The respiration rate measured while sitting, standing, after 50 steps, supine and after 50 skipping are recorded to be ……………, ………………….., ……………………., ……………………… and ……………….. respectively.

Experiment No.: 24

Recording Pulse Oxygen

Objective:	To record the pulse oxygen using pulse oximeter.
Equipment/ Glassware Required:	Pulse oximeter

Principle

It is the way of measuring arterial oxygen saturation level by placing the instrument on periphery. Various peripheral sites are selected such as fingertip, earlobe, forehead, chest, infant foot i.e. a thin part of the body which have higher rate of flow of blood. The principle of the device involves use of two wavelength lights and photodetector. The change in absorbance at different wavelengths is detected by a sensor fitted in the body of photodetector.

Therefore it is a noninvasive method of measuring the oxygen saturation in blood. These instruments are used for diagnosis of COVID-19, change in skin colors, COPD, anemia, hypoxia, obstructive sleep apnea and level of pigmentation.

Following is the blood oxygen levels chart using pulse oxymetry;

Condition	SpO2 Range
Normal	95% to 100%
'Concerning' Blood Oxygen Levels	91 to 95%
Low blood oxygen levels	$\geq 90\%$
Low oxygen saturation affecting brain	80-85%
Cyanosis	Below 67%

Procedure

1. Take the pulse oximeter and switch it on.

2. Place it on the tip of the finger and wait for some time.

3. Look for the readings and record it.

4. For adults, the normal range of oxygen saturation is 95-100%, the range of 93-95% is considered to be mild hypoxia (due to exertion), below 93% value of oxygen saturation is considered to be low oxygen saturation of hypoxic condition and need external oxygen support.

5. The higher oxygen saturation is rare to be found but if it occurs, respiratory alkalosis may occur.

Observation: We learned the importance of maintaining the blood oxygen and carbon dioxide and its methods of determination using pulse oximeter.

Left hand fingers		Right hand fingers		Interpretation
Finger	**SpO2**	**Finger**	**SpO2**	
Finger 1		Finger 1		
Finger 2		Finger 2		
Finger 3		Finger 3		
Finger 4		Finger 4		

Result: The oxygen saturation level in left and right hand finger tips are measured to be: ....

Experiment No: 25

Record Forced Expiratory Volume

Objective:	To record force of air expelled using Peak Flow Meter
Equipment/ Glassware Required:	Peak flow meter

Principle

A peak flow meter is a instrument that measures the peak expiratory flow rate (PEFR). The PEFR is defined as the amount of air a person can quickly force out of their lungs in one breath. The PEFR measurements is used as a guide for managing asthma symptoms.

However, doctors may also recommend peak flow measurements for people with chronic obstructive pulmonary disease (COPD) to determine an increase in symptoms. The normal peak flow is 450-550 L /min in adult males and it is 320-470 L/min in adult females.

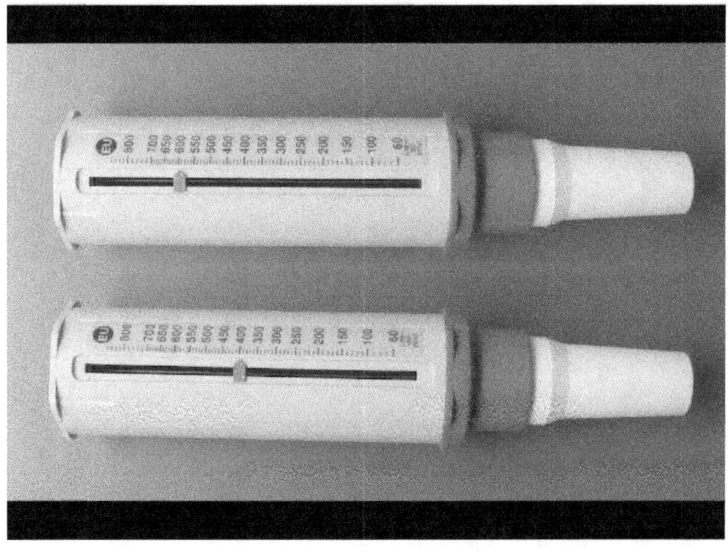

LUNG VOLUMES & CAPACITIES

- Tidal Volume (VT): The volume of air entering the nose or mouth per breath (500 ml).
- Residual Volume (RV): The volume of air left in the lungs after a maximal forced expiration (1.5L).
- Expiratory Reserve Volume (ERV): The volume of air that is expelled from the lung during a maximal forced expiration that starts at the end of normal tidal expiration (1.5L).
- Inspiratory Reserve Volume (IRV): The volume of air that is inhaled into the lung during a maximal forced inspiration starting at the end of a normal tidal inspiration (2.5L).
- Functional Residual Capacity (FRC): the volume of air remaining in the lungs at the end of a normal tidal expiration (3 L).
- Inspiratory Capacity (IC): The volume of air that is inhaled into the lung during a maximal forced inspiration effort that begins at the end of a normal tidal expiration (VT+IRV=3L).
- Vital Capacity (VC): The volume of air that is expelled from the lung during a maximal forced expiration effort starting after a maximal forced inspiration (4.5L).
- Total Lung Capacity (TLC): The volume of air that is inhaled into the lung after a maximal inspiration effort (5-6 L).

Procedure

1. Make sure that the indicator or pointer is set to zero.
2. Stand up straight and take a deep breath for fill your lungs and take a deep breath.
3. Put the flow meter in the mouth with the tongue down, out of the way of the mouthpiece, and close the lips around the mouthpiece.
4. In a single blow, blow out hard and fast. The indicator will move in response to the exhalation.
5. Check the number on the scale next to the pointer or indicator. This is the peak expiratory flow.
6. If you coughed or did not do the steps in correct way, do not write down the number. Instead, do the steps over again
7. Move the indicator back to zero and repeat twice more.
8. Record the best of the three attempts in a chart or notebook.

Observation: We learned the principle and procedure involved in Forced expiratory volume in first second, forced expiratory volume and interpretation of peak flow rate signals.

	Reference Range	Your results	Inference
Forced Expiratory Volume in First Second (FEV1)	Equal or above 80% - Normal Mild - 70-79% Moderate - 60-69% Severe - less than 60%		
Forced Expiratory Volume (FEV)	Equal or above 80% - Normal Mild - 70-79% Moderate - 60-69% Severe - less than 60%		
FEV1/FEV	Equal or above 70% - Normal Mild - 60-69% Moderate - 50-59% Severe - less than 50%		
Color Zone	Green (80-100%) – Normal Yellow (50-80%) – Caution Red (<50%) – Medical alert		

Result: My forced expiratory volume in first second is ...., forced expiratory volume is .... FEV1/FEV is .... and peak flow rate signals is ....

Experiment No.: 26

Measure Body Mass Index

Objective:	To measure height, weight, and BMI
Equipment/ Glassware Required:	Meter scale, weighing balance

Principle

The height and weight of the person defines the body stature. The BMI (body mass index) is defined as measure of relative mass based on the weight and height of the individual. It is commonly used as a screening tool to identify potential weight problems in adults. The formula for the calculation of BMI is -
$$BMI = \frac{mass(kg)}{(height(meter))^2}$$

The alternate way of calculating the BMI is use of nomograph that display height and weight on perpendicular axes and then assign BMI values to colour coded regions.

BMI is grossly used in categorizing an individual as underweight, normal weight, overweight, obese and morbidly obese. Obese and morbidly obese are computed to have higher risk for cardiovascular complications.

BMI CATEGORIES

Category	BMI (kg/m^2)
Underweight (Severe thinness)	< 16.0
Underweight (Moderate thinness)	16.0 – 16.9
Underweight (Mild thinness)	17.0 – 18.4
Normal range	18.5 – 24.9
Overweight (Pre-obese)	25.0 – 29.9
Obese (Class I)	30.0 – 34.9
Obese (Class II)	35.0 – 39.9
Obese (Class III)	≥ 40.0

Height (m) ⟶

Weight (kg)	1.40	1.45	1.50	1.55	1.60	1.65	1.70	1.75	1.80	1.85	1.90	1.95	2.00	2.05	2.10	2.15	2.20
140	71.4	66.6	62.2	58.3	54.7	51.4	48.4	45.7	43.2	40.9	38.8	36.8	35.0	33.3	31.7	30.3	28.9
135	68.9	64.2	60.0	56.2	52.7	49.6	46.7	44.1	41.7	39.4	37.4	35.5	33.8	32.1	30.6	29.2	27.9
130	66.3	61.8	57.8	54.1	58.8	47.8	45.0	42.4	40.1	38.0	36.0	34.2	32.5	30.9	29.5	28.1	26.9
125	63.8	59.5	55.6	52.0	48.8	45.9	43.3	40.8	38.6	36.5	34.6	32.9	31.3	29.7	28.3	27.0	25.8
120	61.2	57.1	53.3	49.9	46.9	44.1	41.5	39.2	37.0	35.1	33.2	31.6	30.0	28.6	27.2	26.0	24.8
115	58.7	54.7	51.1	47.9	44.9	42.2	39.8	37.6	35.5	33.6	31.9	30.2	28.8	27.4	26.1	24.9	23.8
110	56.1	52.3	48.9	45.8	43.0	40.4	38.1	35.9	34.0	32.1	30.5	28.9	27.5	26.2	24.9	23.8	22.7
105	53.6	49.9	46.7	43.7	41.0	38.6	36.3	34.3	32.4	30.7	29.1	27.6	26.3	25.0	23.8	22.7	21.7
100	51.0	47.9	44.4	41.6	39.1	36.7	34.6	32.7	30.9	29.2	27.7	26.3	25.0	23.8	22.7	21.6	20.7
95	48.5	45.2	42.2	39.5	37.1	34.9	32.9	31.0	29.3	27.8	26.3	25.0	23.8	22.6	21.5	20.6	19.6
90	45.9	42.8	40.0	37.2	35.2	33.1	31.1	29.4	27.8	26.3	24.9	23.7	22.5	21.4	20.4	19.5	18.6
85	43.4	40.4	37.8	35.4	33.2	31.2	29.4	27.8	26.2	24.8	23.5	22.4	21.3	20.2	19.3	18.4	17.6
80	40.8	38.0	35.6	33.3	31.3	29.4	27.7	26.1	24.7	23.4	22.2	21.0	20.0	19.0	18.1	17.3	16.5
75	38.3	35.7	33.3	31.2	29.3	27.5	26.0	24.5	23.1	21.9	20.8	19.7	18.8	17.8	17.0	16.2	15.5
70	35.7	33.3	31.1	29.1	27.1	25.7	24.2	22.9	21.6	20.5	19.4	18.4	17.5	16.7	15.9	15.1	14.5
65	33.2	30.9	28.9	27.1	25.4	23.9	22.5	21.2	20.1	19.0	18.0	17.1	16.3	15.5	14.7	14.1	13.4
60	30.6	28.5	26.7	25.0	23.4	22.0	20.8	19.6	18.5	17.5	16.6	15.8	15.0	14.3	13.6	13.0	12.4
55	28.1	26.2	24.4	22.9	21.5	20.2	19.0	18.0	17.0	16.1	15.2	14.5	13.8	13.1	12.5	11.9	11.4
50	25.5	23.8	22.2	20.8	19.5	18.4	17.3	16.3	15.4	14.6	13.9	13.1	12.5	11.9	11.3	10.8	10.3

☐ Underweight   ☐ Normal Weight   ☐ Overweight

☐ Obese (Class I)   ☐ Obese (Class II)   ☐ Obese (Class III)

Procedure

1. Using a meter scale, measure the height of the subject and record it.

2. Now using the weighing balance, measure the weight of the subject and record it.

3. Now convert the height recorded into meters and recorded weight in kilograms.

4. Now using the given formula, calculate the BMI.

5. Alternately, use the nomogram and point out the recorded values of height and weight on the chart followed by the determination of corresponding BMI value.

Observation: Following are my details and my friends:

Sl No	Name of subject	Height	Weight	BMI	Interpretation
1					
2					
3					

Result: Based on above observation BMI of my friend was calculated to be
………………..

Based on it we conclude that my friend is ………………….

Experiment No: 27

Cardiovascular System

Objective:	To study the human cardiovascular system with the help of chart, models, and specimens
Equipment/ Glassware Required:	Chart/model/specimen of human cardiovascular system

Principle

The circulatory system, commonly referred to as the cardiovascular system, is made up of the heart and a closed system of veins, arteries, and capillaries. The CVS is responsible for the transportation of blood throughout the body. As the blood carries several substances like oxygen, food, hormones etc. to body cells it becomes very crucial system for body.

Heart: The first size heart acts as the pumping organ and vessels serves as the pipeline for the blood. It is situated in the mediastinum cavity of the thorax and weighs 250–350 g. There are two chambers on the left side and two on the right side, making up its four chambers. It performs mechanical, motor, and electrical tasks. The endocardium is the inner membrane, while the pericardium is the outermost layer covering the heart.

Chambers of the heart: The heart is divided by septa, or partitions, into right and left halves, and each half is subdivided into two chambers. The interventricular septum divides the lower chambers, the ventricles, from the higher chambers, the atria, which are separated by the interatrial septum. The atria receive blood from various parts of the body and pass it into the ventricles. The ventricles, in turn, pump blood to the lungs and to the remainder of the body. Tricuspid and bicuspid valves, respectively, divide the right and left side ventricles from the atrium. The cardiac valves ensure the unidirectional flow of blood.

Location of the heart: It has a cone-like shape, with the wide base pointing rightward and upward and the tip pointing leftward and downward. It is situated in the thoracic cavity of the chest, above the diaphragm (the muscular partition between the chest and abdominal cavities), behind the sternum (breastbone), in front of the oesophagus, descending aorta, trachea (windpipe), between lungs. The heart is positioned to the left of the midline by about two thirds.

Wall of the heart: The wall of the heart consists of three distinct layers—the epicardium (outer layer), the myocardium (middle layer), and the endocardium (inner layer). Coronary vessels supplying arterial blood to the heart penetrate the epicardium before entering the myocardium. The thickness of the myocardium varies according to the pressure generated to move blood to its destination. The myocardium of the left ventricle, which must drive blood out into the systemic circulation, is, therefore, thickest; the myocardium of the right ventricle, which propels blood to the lungs, is moderately thickened, while the atrial walls are relatively thin.

Coronary circulation: The circulation of blood to meet the metabolic demand of the heart is called coronary circulation. The coronary arteries provide an intermittent supply of blood to the heart, predominantly when the heart is relaxed (during diastole), as the entrance to the coronary arteries is open at that point of the cardiac cycle. The venous drainage system of the heart uses the coronary veins, which follow a course similar to that of the coronary arteries. The coronary sinus is a collection of coronary veins (small, middle, great and oblique veins, left marginal vein and left posterior ventricular vein) that drain into the RA at the posterior aspect of the heart. Two thirds of the cardiac venous blood is returned to the heart via the coronary sinus, while one third is returned directly into the heart (with the anterior cardiac veins opening directly into the RA and the smallest coronary veins into all four chambers).

Sinoatrial Node: In the heart, the electrical changes needed to generate a cardiac impulse are regulated by its own conduction system, which starts with a sequence of excitation in sinoatrial node (SAN), situated in the right atrium. This is the heart's natural pacemaker. When working properly, it sets the heart rhythm (sinus rhythm) and initiates impulses that act on the myocardium, stimulating cardiac contraction.

Atrioventricular Node: The cardiac impulse passes from the SAN into the atria, which starts to contract, and the impulse is transmitted to another mass of specialised cells, the atrioventricular node (AVN). The AVN is situated in the inter-atrial septum, a band of tissue between the RA and LA that provides a pathway of conduction between the atria and the ventricles. There is a slight delay (of 0.1 seconds) of the impulse at the AVN because the fibres of the AVN are smaller, which gives the atria time to contract and empty into the ventricles before ventricular contraction occurs.

Bundle of His: The impulse then travels down into a large bundle of specialised tissue, the Bundle of His, which conducts it down the ventricles.

The Bundle of His subsequently splits into the right and left bundles in the interventricular septum.

Purkinje fibres: Purkinje fibres then continue down to the inferior aspect of the heart, before looping upwards and travelling in the lateral aspects of the RV and LV.

Blood vessels: are categorized into arteries and veins. Arteries carry oxygenated blood from heart to peripheral organs. Whereas the veins carry deoxygenated blood from peripheral organs to heart. Veins have larger diameter with valves to prevent backflow. Blood vessels also remove carbon dioxide and other waste.

Procedure

Follow the below given steps:

1. Collect chart, specimen and models of human cardiovascular system
2. Observe different parts of heart
3. Identify the difference between arteries and veins
4. Understand the location and direction of heart
5. Use model to identify SA node, AV node and fibres
6. Differentiate bicuspid and tricuspid valve
7. Observe the cardiopulmonary circulation of blood
8. Understand the branching process of arteries
9. Draw the neat labelled diagram
10. Record your observation

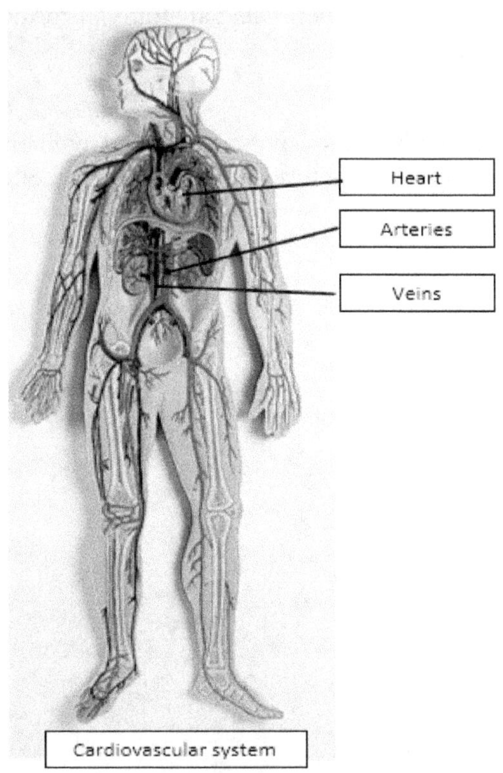

Heart
Arteries
Veins
Cardiovascular system

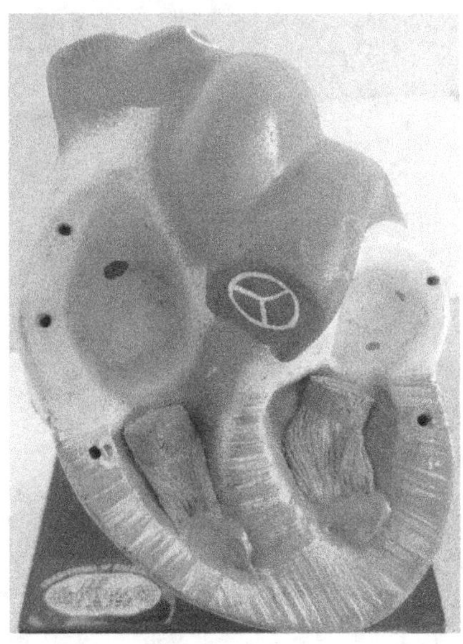

Observation: We learned the theory and anatomy of cardiovascular system using chart and models.

Result: Cardiovascular system has been studied with the help of chart, models, and specimens. The pictures are drawn and labelled.

Experiment No.: 28

Respiratory System

Objective:	To study the respiratory system with the help of chart, models, and specimens
Equipment/ Glassware Required:	Chart/model/specimen of respiratory system

Principle

Respiratory system is the network of organs and tissues that help you breathe. This system helps your body absorb oxygen from the air so that your organs can work. It also cleans waste gases, such as carbon dioxide, from your blood. The respiratory system is present in the thoracic cavity. It consists of nostrils, nasal cavity, larynx, pharynx, trachea, lungs, bronchi, etc.

The exchange of gases between the blood and the lunges is called as external respiration while that between the blood and the body cells is referred as internal respiration.

It includes the following organs.

Nose: It is the first organ of the respiratory system and consists of two large irregular cavities and also contains muscles secreting goblet cells.

Function

- The air is warmed as it passes over the surface of the nose.
- It is moistened by contact with the moist mucous.
- Air is filtered as dust particles bacteria stick to the mucous.
- Nose is the organ of sense of smell

Pharynx: It is a tube 12 to 14 cm in length. It starts from the base of the skull up to the sixth cervical vertebra. It lies behind the nose, the mouth, the larynx. It is wider at its upper end. It is lined by mucous membrane. It has three parts nasopharynx, oropharynx and laryngopharynx.

Function: It is an organ involved in both respiratory and digestive function.

Larynx: It is called as `voice box`. It starts from the root of the tongue and the hyoid bone up to the trachea. It lies at the level of 3rd, 4th, 5th, and 6th cervical vertebra. There is little difference in the size of the larynx until the puberty. After puberty it grows larger in male.

Function: It provides a passage way for air between the pharynx and the trachea.

Trachea: It is also referred as wind pipe. It is a continuation of larynx. It extends up to the level of the 5th thoracic vertebra. At this level it bifurcates into the right and left bronchus which enters into each lung. It lies in median plane in front of oesophagus and is about 11 cm in length. It is composed of 16-20 incomplete `C` shaped rings situated one above the other and made up of hyaline cartilage composed of fibrous tissue, elastic tissue, connective tissue and ciliated columnar tissue.

Bronchi: The two bronchi start at the level of 5th thoracic vertebra. The right bronchus is wider, shorter tube as compared to the left bronchus. The right bronchus is 2.5 cm in length while the left bronchus is 5 cm in length. After entering in the right lung, the right bronchus divides in two branches. One of which goes to each lobes of the lung. Each branch then divides and subdivides into smaller branches. Bronchi are lined with ciliated columnar epithelium.

Bronchioles: The air passage without the cartilage in their walls are referred as `bronchioles`. The minute bronchiole which further divides to form alveolar ducts leads to sac like structure called as alveoli. These are responsible for exchange of gases.

Lungs: Lungs are in two in number. They lie on each side of the midline in the thoracic cavity. Lungs are cone shaped and show apex, base costal surface, and medial surface. The right lungs is divided into three parts- superior, middle, inferior while left lungs is divided into two parts –superior and inferior. The lungs are composed of bronchi, smaller air passage, alveoli, connective tissues blood vessel and nerves. Lungs are responsible for exchange of gases.

Procedure

Collect chart, specimen and models of respiratory system

- Observe different parts of respiratory system
- Identify nose, pharynx, larynx, trachea

- Recognize the branching of trachea, and the number of lobes in the lungs.

- Differentiate the role of nose, pharynx, trachea, lungs

- Draw the neat labelled diagram

- Record your observation

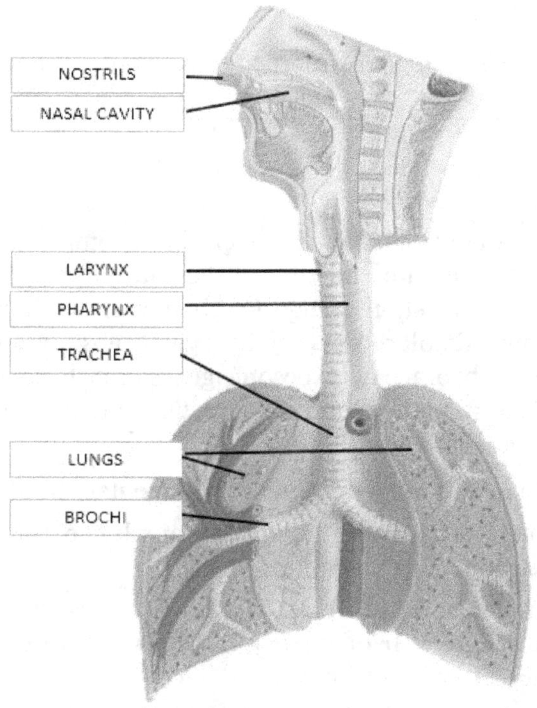

Observation: We learned the theory and anatomy of respiratory system using chart and models.

Result: Respiratory system has been studied with the help of chart, models, and specimens. The pictures are drawn and labelled.

Experiment No.: 29

Digestive System

Objective:	To study the digestive system with the help of chart, models, and specimens
Equipment/ Glassware Required:	Chart/model/specimen of digestive system

Principle

The digestive system in human is present in abdominal region of human body. It starts from mouth and ends at the anus. The digestive system is responsible for the digestion of ingested food, it breaks down the complex food materials into simpler forms and helps in its absorption too. It consists of organs like mouth, oral cavity, oesophagus, stomach, pancreas, liver, gall bladder, small intestine, large intestine, rectum and anus. The activities of the alimentary canal are grouped as:

  (i) Ingestion means taking of food into alimentary tract

  (ii) Digestion means break down of complex particles into simple absorbable one

  (iii) Absorption means the process by which the digested food substance passes through wall of organs of alimentary canal into blood for circulation all over the body.

  (iv) Elimination means food substance which have been eaten but cannot be digested and absorbed are excreted by the bowel as faces

Tongue

It is made up of three elements epithelium, muscles and glands. It shows taste buds and papillae. It is voluntary muscular structure which occupies the floor of the mouth cavity. It serves the following functions---

(a) Mastication (chewing)

(b) Deglutition (swallowing)

(c) Taste (general sensation)

(d) Speech (essential for speech)

(e) Secretion (mucus and serous fluids)

Teeth: Teeth are embedded in the socket of the alveolar ridges of the mandible and maxilla. It exists in two forms- temporary teeth (20), and permanent teeth (32). The permanent teeth show molars, premolars, incisors and canine. Molar and premolars are used for girding and chewing food while incisor and canine helps in cutting or biting of pieces of food

Pharynx: The pharyngeal and laryngeal parts of the pharynx are involved in the digestive system. Food from oral cavity passes to the pharynx and then to the esophagus. The pharynx has both respiratory and digestive functions.

Esophagus: It is first organ system and is about 25 cm long. It is continuous with the pharynx above and joins the stomach below the diaphragm. It receives the food from the pharynx and passes to the stomach by series of peristaltic contractions.

Stomach: It is J shaped dilated portion of the alimentary tract. It is present in the epigastric, umbilical, hypochondriac region of the abdominal cavity. The principal anatomic regions of the stomach are the cardia, fundus, body, and pylorus. Stomach play important role in the digestive system.

 (i)   It receives food material and act as a reservoir of food.

 (ii)   The movement of stomach helps in proper mixing with digestive juices and helps to propel the food into duodenum.

 (iii)   It secretes gastric juices which act as digestive fluid. The hydrochloric acid of the gastric juices act as antiseptic against swallowed bacteria.

 (iv)   It absorbs small quantities of water, saline, alcohol, glucose and certain drugs.

Small Intestine: It is about 5 meter in length. It extends from the pyloric sphincter to the ileocecal sphincter. It lies in abdominal cavity surrounded by large intestine. It is described in three parts- (i) the duodenum which is the first part and is about 25 cm in length and `C` shaped. It has common opening for the pancreatic and bile duct. (ii) The jejunum is the middle part. (iii) The ileum is the terminal part. Small intestine is the main site where complete digestion of food occurs. Mechanical digestion in the small intestine involves segmentation and migrating motility complexes. Absorption occurs via diffusion, facilitated diffusion, osmosis, and active transport; most absorption occurs in the small intestine.

Large Intestine: It is about 1.5meter longs. It extends from the ileocecal sphincter to the anus. It includes the cecum, colon, rectum, and anal canal. It surrounds small intestine. Functions of large intestine are:

(i)   Absorption of water, ions, vitamins and drugs.

(ii) Large number of micro-organism are present in it e.g. *E. coli* which helps in the synthesis of vitamins.

(iii) It is involved in the act of defecation.

Accessory organ of digestive system:

Salivary glands: Three pairs of salivary glands are:

(1) parotid,

(2) submandibular

(3) lingual.

These glands pour their secretion into mouth. The saliva serves the following functions: (i) it keeps mouth moist (ii) it dilutes hot and irritant substance and prevents the injury to mucous membrane (iii) it helps in process of mastication of the food stuff and in preparing it into a bolus, suitable for deglutition. (iv) constant flow of saliva washes down the food debris and thus prevents the growth of the bacteria (v) Maltose in the saliva converts into glucose.

Liver: it is the largest gland of the body which weighs about 1-2.3 kg. Bile is secretory as well as excretory product of liver. It involved in following function.

(i) Carbohydrate, lipid and protein metabolism

(ii) Converts glucose to glycogen in presence of insulin

(iii) It stores vitamins and minerals

(iv) Excretion of bilirubin

(v) Activation of vitamin D

(vi) Phagocytosis

(vii) Excretion of bilirubin.

Pancreas: it is pale grey gland weighs about 60 gms. It is present in epigastric region of abdominal cavity; it secretes pancreatic juice which is involved in chemical digestion of food

Procedure

Collect chart, specimen and models of digestive system

- Observe different parts of digestive system

- Identify mouth, pharynx, oesophagus, stomach, small intestine, large intestine, liver, and pancreas

- Recognize different parts of stomach and small intestine.
- Differentiate the role of salivary glands, liver, pancreas.
- Draw the neat labelled diagram
- Record your observation

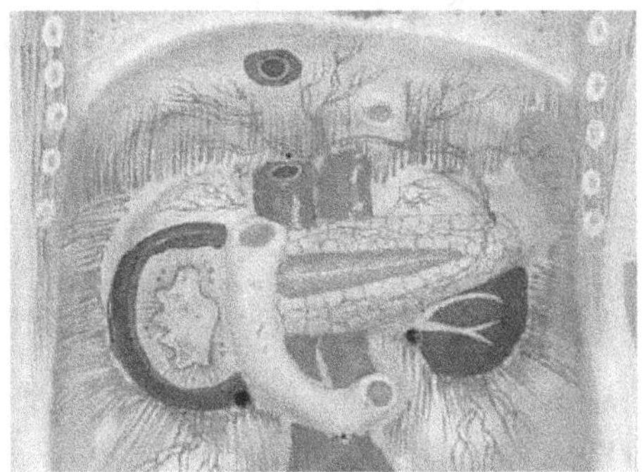

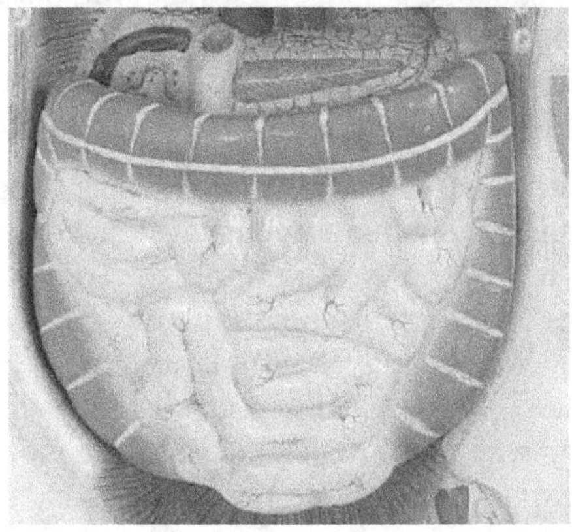

Observation: We learned the theory and anatomy of digestive system using chart and models.

Result: Digestive system has been studied with the help of chart, models, and specimens. The pictures are drawn and labelled.

Experiment No.: 30

Study of Human Nervous System

Objective:	To study the human nervous system with the help of chart, models, and specimens
Equipment/ Glassware Required:	Chart/model/specimen of human nervous system

Principle

It is complex system involved in conducting impulses from one part of the body to other and vice versa. Nerves are fibres and arranged in cylindrical form originating in brain and spinal cord branching out to different parts of the body. The neurons a structural and functional unit are arranged similar to electrical wires. Neurons conduct stimuli from receptors to the spinal cord and brain. The brain consists of 100 trillion neuronal connections.

Classification of nervous system: The system has two major parts central nervous system and peripheral nervous system. The sensory neurons, nerves and ganglia are the parts of peripheral nervous system connecting one another. Further based on its functions peripheral nervous system is divided into somatic or voluntary and autonomic or involuntary nervous system. The somatic nervous system connects the brain and spinal cord to muscles and sensory receptors in the skin. The autonomic nervous system involved in regulating self-controlled physiologic and metabolic functions such as BP, Heart rate, and endocrine functions.

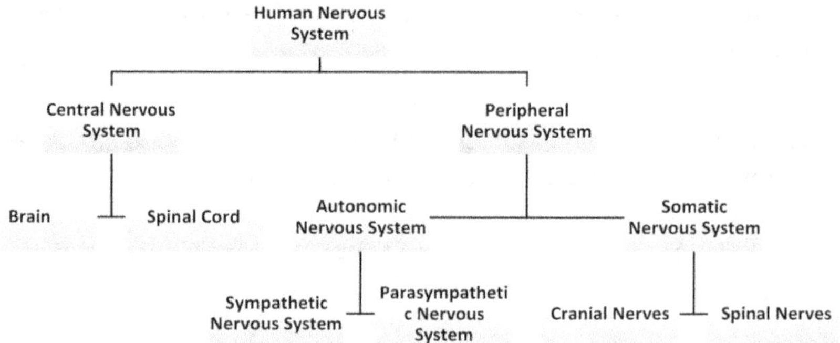

Brain and parts: The brain and spinal cord are the parts of central nervous system and are derived from the embryonic neural tube. The cerebrospinal fluid a clear nourishing fluid floats in both brain and spinal cord. Both of them are covered by a protective membrane called meninges. The bony layer covering approximate 1500 g of the brain is called neurocranium and spinal cord is present in vertebral column. The glial cells present in brain are known to support, nourish and protect nerve cells. The brain is majorly divided into three parts; cerebrum, brain stem and cerebellum. The brainstem consists of medulla oblongata, midbrain, pons, epithalamus, hypothalamus, thalamus, subthalamus and pons.

Neurons: Neurons are the longest cells of the body having three parts dendrites, body and axons. Signals are received through dendrites and send through axons. Neurotransmission process involves the release of chemicals or neurotransmitters at synapses for signal transmission. Neurons covered by myelin sheath are called myelinated neurons and neurons not covered by myelin sheath are called non-myelinated neurons.

Diseases of Nervous System: There are several common neurological diseases diagnosed and reported few of the important diseases or disorders includes epilepsy, multiple sclerosis, amyotrophic lateral sclerosis, Alzheimer's disease, Pankinson's disease, meningitis, encephalitis, etc.

Procedure

Follow the below given steps:

1. Collect chart, specimen and models of human nervous system
2. Observe different parts of brain and study their functions
3. Identify cranial nerves
4. Recognize neuronal synapses
5. Differentiate presynaptic and postsynaptic neurons
6. Study structure of neuron and study their functions
7. Observe the structure of spinal cord and identify cervical, thoracic and lumbar regions.
8. Draw the neat labelled diagram of brain and neuron
9. Record your observation

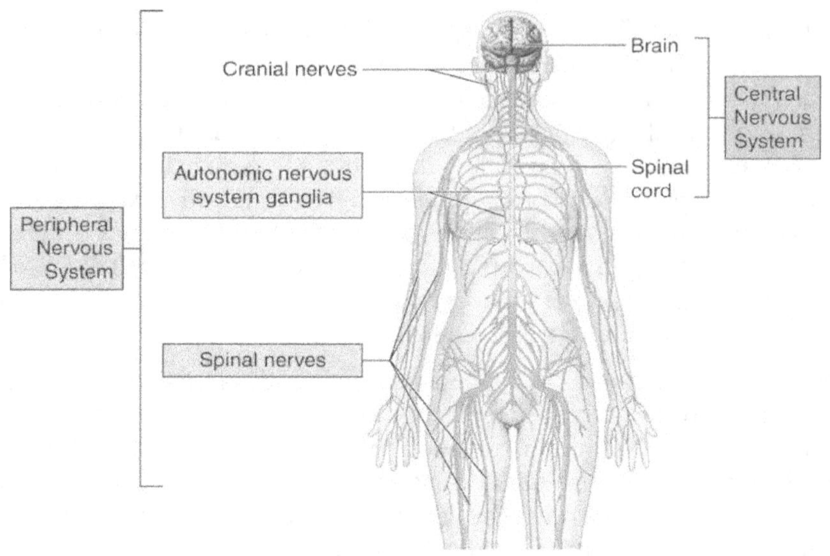

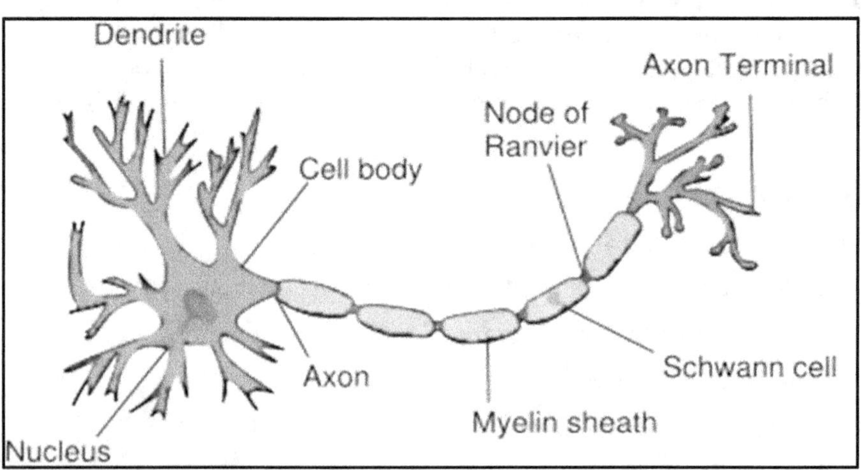

Observation: We learned the theory and anatomy of nervous system using chart and models.

Result: Nervous system has been studied with the help of chart, models, and specimens. The pictures are drawn and labelled.

Experiment No.: 31

Urinary System

Objective:	To study the urinary system with the help of chart, models, and specimens
Equipment/ Glassware Required:	Chart/model/specimen of urinary system

Principle

The body takes nutrients from food and changes them to energy. After the body has taken the food components that it needs, waste products are left behind in the bowel and in the blood. The kidney and urinary systems help the body to get rid of liquid waste called urea. They also help to keep chemicals (such as potassium and sodium) and water in balance. Urea is produced when foods containing protein (such as meat, poultry, and certain vegetables) are broken down in the body. Urea is carried in the blood to the kidneys. This is where it is removed, along with water and other wastes in the form of urine. The kidneys have other important functions. They control blood pressure and produce the hormone erythropoietin. This hormone controls red blood cell production in the bone marrow. The kidneys also control the acid-base balance and conserve fluids. The urinary system in the human body is present in the lower abdomen. The urinary system is also known as excretory system and it consist of organs like kidney, ureter, urinary bladder and urethra. The various parts of this system are as follows:

Kidney: These are two in number. They lie on the posterior wall of abdomen. It lies on each side of the vertebral column. The Kidney extends from the level of twelfth thoracic vertebra to the third lumber vertebra. The right kidney is slightly lower than the left kidney. The left kidney is slightly narrower and longer than the right kidney. Each kidney is bean shaped and is about 11 cm. long, 6 cm wide and 3 cm. thick. The renal fat encloses each kidney. The two kidneys together contain about 2,400,000 nephrons, and each nephron is capable of forming urine. It maintains the normal composition of the plasma through the elimination of excess water and waste products of protein metabolism. It also play important role in regulation of acid base balance of the body.

Ureters: These are the two tubes conveying the urine from kidney to the urinary bladder. Each ureter is continuous with the funnel shaped pelvis of the kidney. Each tube measures about 25 to 30 cm. in length. The diameter of each tube is 3 mm. Each ureter passes downwards through the abdominal cavity and opens into posterior aspect of the base of the urinary bladder. It propels the urine from the kidney to the bladder.

Urinary bladder: It lies in the pelvic cavity. It is roughly pear shaped. The bladder opens into urethra. The urinary bladder act as a reservoir for the urine when approximately 200-300ml of urine accumulates in bladder. This stimulates the autonomic nerve endings within the membrane wall of the bladder wall. Micturation occurs when the muscular wall of the bladder contracts, the internal sphincter dilates and the external sphincter relaxes.

Urethra: It is a canal which extends from the neck of bladder to the exterior. Its size depends upon the gender. The female urethra is 4 cm. in length approx. It opens into the external urethral orifice just in front of vagina. The male urethra is about 15- 20cm in length, it conducts the urine from the urinary bladder to pass out of the body.

Procedure: Follow the below given steps:

1. Collect chart, specimen and models of urinary system

2. Observe different parts of urinary system

3. Identify renal artery, renal vein, layers of tissue surrounding kidney, internal regions of kidney, urinary bladder, urethra

4. Recognize the shape and structure of kidney, urinary bladder, length of urethra

5. Differentiate between the functions of different parts of urinary system

6. Draw the neat labelled diagram

7. Record your observation

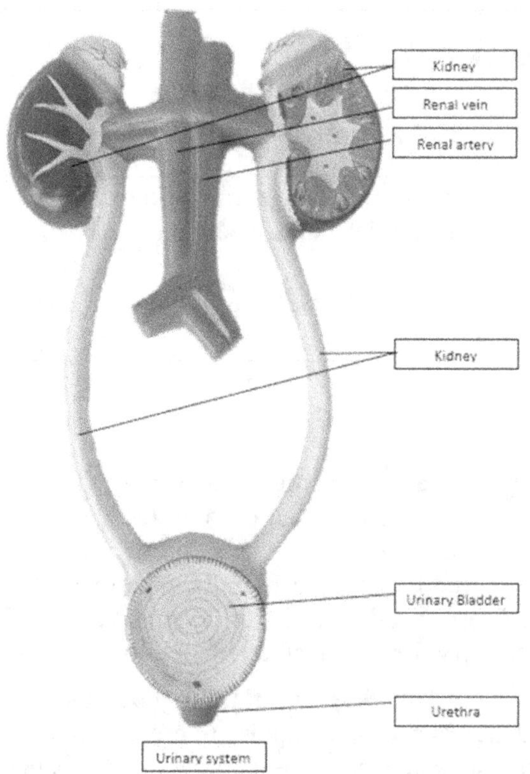

Observation: We learned the theory and anatomy of urinary system using chart and models.

Result: Urinary system has been studied with the help of chart, models, and specimens. The pictures are drawn and labelled.

Experiment No.: 32

Endocrine System

Objective:	To study the human endocrine system with the help of chart, models, and specimens
Equipment/ Glassware Required:	Chart/model/specimen of human endocrine system

Principle

It is well known that the body homeostasis is maintained by the endocrine system and nervous system through long term and shortterm effects respectively. The endocrine system acts through secretion of chemicals called hormones directly into the blood for actions on different organs and/or systems. These glands are also known as ductless glands as they do not have ducts to carry them to surface for action.

The endocrine system is present throughout the human body, like pituitary, hypothalamaus, pineal glands are present in brain region; thyroid and parathyroid glands in neck region; adrenal gland, pancreas gland, testis and ovaries in the abdominal and pelvic region. Each endocrine has specific secretion and function to perform.

The hormones secreted by endocrine glands are involved in controlling and coordinating body's metabolism, energy level, reproduction, growth and development, and response to injury, stress, and mood. The following are integral parts of the endocrine system:

Hypothalamus. It is located at the base of the brain and involved in regulating activities of pituitary gland. Its main function is to regulate body temperature, appetite, thirst, sleep and blood pressure.

Pineal body. It is located in the middle of brain and secrets melatonin to regulate circadian rhythm.

Pituitary. It is also known as master gland as it controls many functions of the body and other endocrine glands.

Thyroid and parathyroid. The thyroid and parathyroid glands are located below the larynx and secrets thyroid and parathyroid hormones for regulating metabolic activities and calcium balance.

Adrenal. These are located on the top of each kidney. They secret adrenaline, noradrenaline, glucocorticoids and mineralocorticoids to maintain blood pressure and regulate metabolism.

Pancreas. It is located behind the stomach and secrets insulin and glucagon for regulating the level of blood sugar.

Ovary. These glands are located on the sides of the uterus secreting estrogen and progesterone required for female reproduction.

Testis. A pair of male glands present in a pouch hanging outside the body and secrets testosterone and sperm responsible for male reproduction.

Procedure

Follow the below given steps:

1. Collect chart, specimen and models of endocrine system
2. Observe different locations of glands in the body
3. Identify hypothalamus located on the base of brain
4. Recognize pancreas located in abdomen
5. Differentiate thyroid and parathyroid gland
6. Locate the presence of adrenal glands on top of the kidney
7. Differentiate structure and function of male and female glands
8. Draw the neat labelled diagram
9. Record your observation

Observation: We learned the theory and anatomy of endocrine system using chart and models.

Result: Human endocrine system has been studied with the help of chart, models, and specimens. The pictures are drawn and labelled.

Experiment No: 33

Human Reproductive System

Objective:	To study the human reproductive system with the help of chart, models, and specimens
Equipment/ Glassware Required:	Chart/model/specimen of male and female human reproductive system

Principle

The reproductive systems of human body are different for male and female. Reproductive system is responsible for the function of reproduction in humans. In both, males and females, the reproductive system is present in the lower abdomen and pelvic region of the body.

The male reproductive system includes the testis, ductus epididymis, ductus deferens, ejaculatory duct, urethra, seminal vesicles, prostate, Cowper's glands, and penis, which are as follows: -

Scrotum: It is a pouch of deeply pigmented skin. It hangs from the root of the penis and consists of loose skin and superficial fascia. It is divided into two parts and each part contains one testis.

Testis: These are male reproductive glands which lie in the scrotum. Each testis is composed of 200-300 lobules called as seminiferous tubule, in which sperm cells are made; sertoli cells, which nourish sperm cells and secrete inhibin; and Leydig (interstitial) cells, which produce male sex hormone testosterone. Testis involved in spermatogenesis, and secrets testosterone hormone.

Spermatic cords: These are two in number, one leading from each testis. They suspend testes in scrotum.

Seminal vesicles: It secretes an alkaline, viscous fluid that contains fructose. It constitutes about 60% of the volume of semen and contributes to sperm viability.

Ejaculatory ducts: These are two short tubes, 2cm long and formed by the union of the duct from the seminal vesicle and ampulla of the vas deferens is the passageway for ejection of sperm and secretions of the seminal vesicles in to the first portion of the urethra, the prostatic urethra.

Prostate gland: The secretion of the prostate gland consists of a slightly acidic fluid that constitutes about 60% of volume of semen and contributes to sperm motility.

The bulbourethral (Cowper's) gland: The Cowper's gland secretes mucus for lubrication and an alkaline substance that neutralizes acid.

The female reproductive system consists of vagina, Uterus, Uterine tube or fallopian tube.

Vagina: The vagina is the fibro muscular tube connecting the internal & external organs of generation. It is lined by elastic, alveolar, smooth muscle tissue.

Uterus: The uterus is hollow muscular organ, pear shaped and flat. It is about 7.5 cm long, 5 cm wide 2.5 cm thick and about 30-40 gm. After puberty, uterus undergoes regular cycle of changes which prepares it to receive nourishes and protects a fertilized ovum. During pregnancy walls of the uterus relax to accommodate the growing fetus.

Uterine: The uterine tube lies on each side of the uterus. They are about 10 cm long. The uterine tube conveys the ovum from the ovary to the uterus. Fertilization of the ovum usually takes place in the uterine tubes.

Ovaries: The ovaries are the female sex glands. The length of each ovary is 2.5 cm while the breadth is about 2 cm. while the thickness is about 1 cm. If the ovum is fertilized it embeds in the wall of uterus where it grows and develops. If the ovum is not fertilized the corpus luteum degenerates, menstruation occurs and next cycle begins.

Procedure

Follow the below given steps:

- Collect chart, specimen and models of human reproductive system
- Observe different parts of the male and female reproductive system
- Identify epididymis, testes, penis, seminal vesicle, prostate gland of male reproductive system
- Identify cervix, vagina, uterus, ovary, and fallopian rube of female reproductive system.
- Recognize the difference between male and female reproductive system
- Differentiate prostate gland, Cowper's gland and seminal vesicle

- Draw the neat labelled diagram
- Record your observation

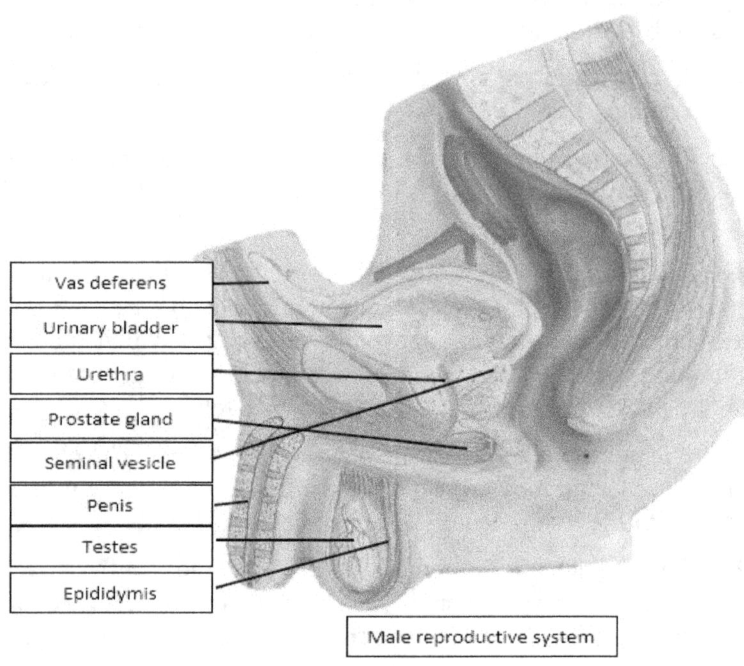

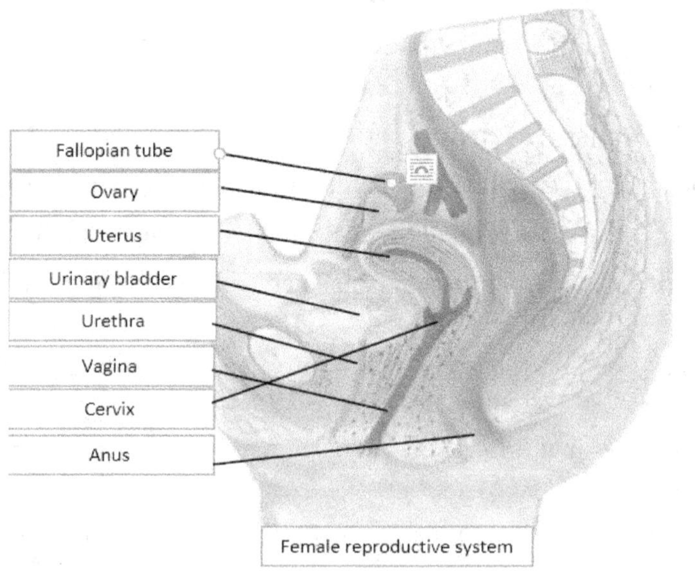

Observation: We learned the theory and anatomy of male and female reproductive system using chart and models.

Result: Male and female reproductive system has been studied with the help of chart, models, and specimens. The pictures are drawn and labelled.

Experiment No.: 34

Eye

Objective:	To study the human eye with the help of chart, models, and specimens
Equipment/ Glassware Required:	Chart/model/specimen of human eye.

Principle

Eye is the most important sensory organ of the human body responsible for the sight and reception of light stimulus. It reacts to visible light and allows us to use visual information for various purposes including seeing things, keeping our balance, and maintaining circadian rhythm. Eyes exist in pair in humans and situated on the left and right side of the face.

Eyes are located in the bony cavities called orbits in the skull. The movement of eyes is controlled by six extraocular muscles. The frontal part of the eye is called anterior segment and behind is called posterior segment. The anterior segment composed of cornea, iris and lens. Whereas the posterior segment is composed of the vitreous, retina, choroid and sclera.

It is an optical device almost spherical in shape. The outermost white part of the eye is called sclera and the innermost layer is the choroid. The clear part of the optical component is called cornea which helps in focusing of light. The pupil is an aperture and colored part of the eye that controls the amount of light passing is called iris. The retina is a part of the optical system where the images fall and are processed and carried to brain via optic nerve. Two different types of cells rods and cones help in visibility under low intensity of light and high intensity of light respectively. They are also responsible for visibility of black-and-white and colored images.

In general the eye is covered with three coats. The outermost layer is called fibrous tunic, the middle layer is called vascular tunic and the innermost layer is called retina. The shape of the lens is controlled by ciliary muscles.

Procedure

Follow the below given steps:

- Collect chart, specimen and models of eye
- Observe different parts of eye
- Identify retina and retinal vessels in the eye
- Recognize cornea and lens
- Identify vitreous, choroid and sclera
- Differentiate yellow spot and blind spot
- Identify pupil and iris
- Recognize aqueous humor and vitreous humor
- Draw the neat labelled diagram
- Record your observation

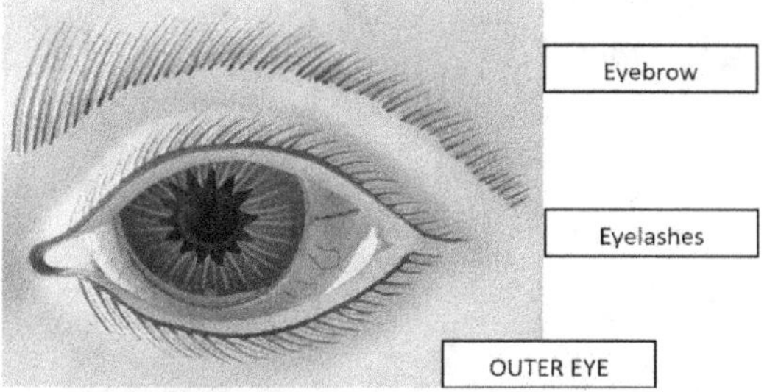

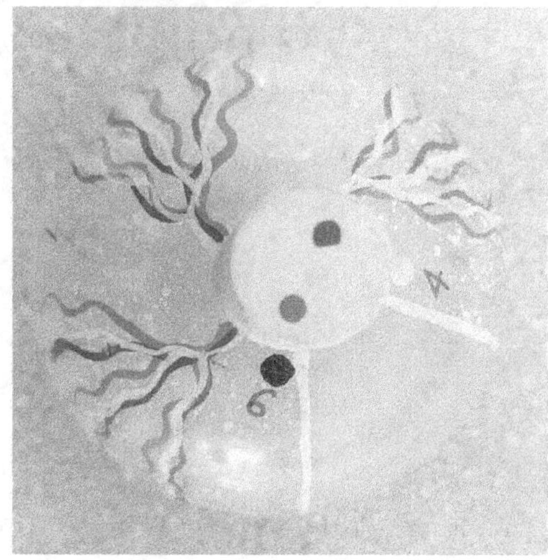

Observation: We learned the theory and anatomy of human eye using chart and models.

Result: Human eye structure has been studied with the help of chart, models, and specimens. The pictures are drawn and labelled.

Experiment No.: 35

Ear

Objective:	To study the human ear with the help of chart, models, and specimens
Equipment/ Glassware Required:	Chart/model/specimen of human ear.

Principle

The ears are the paired organs of human body present on the sides of head region. The ears are responsible for the sensation of sound, postural equilibrium and coordination of head and eye movements. The ears consist of three distinguished parts i.e. outer, middle and inner.

The outer ear consists of auricle or pinna projected from the side of the head, auditory canal and the inner end is closed by tympanic membrane. The pinna is made up of elastic cartilage and covered by skin. The lobule is a fleshy lower part of the auricle containing no cartilage. The function of the outer ear is to collect sound waves and direct them to the tympanic membrane which is of 8-10 mm in diameter. The cerumen or earwax is produced by modified sweat glands to discourage insect from entering the ear.

The middle ear is air filled cavity present in temporal bone. It consists of three small bones the malleus, incus, and stapes, and together they are called the auditory ossicles. These bones are suspended by ligaments so that they freely vibrate and amplify the vibrations received from tympanic membrane and passing them to inner ear.

The inner ear consists of two functional units i.e vestibular apparatus and cochlea. The vestibular apparatus consists of vestibule and semicircular canals containing sensory organs for postural equilibrium and cochlea for hearing. The vestibular nerve innervate these sensory organs and carry the information to brain. The watery fluid filling the labyrinth space is called perilymph.

Procedure

Follow the below given steps:

- Collect chart, specimen and models of ear

- Observe different parts of ear

- Identify Hammer (malleus), Anvil (incus) and Stirrup (stapes) and observe their arrangement.

- Recognize tympanic membrane

- Differentiate external, middle and inner ear

- Draw the neat labelled diagram

- Record your observation

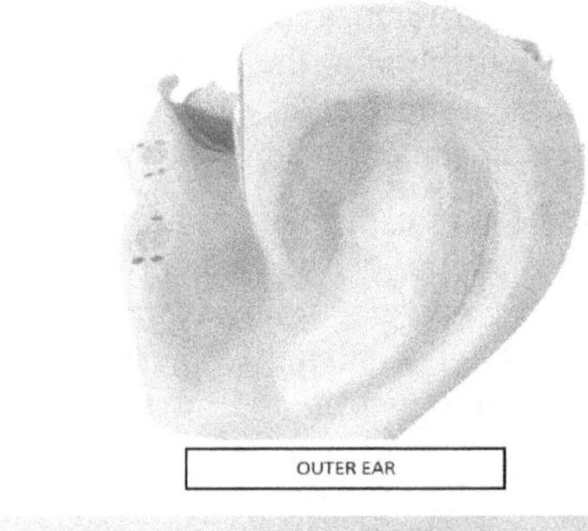

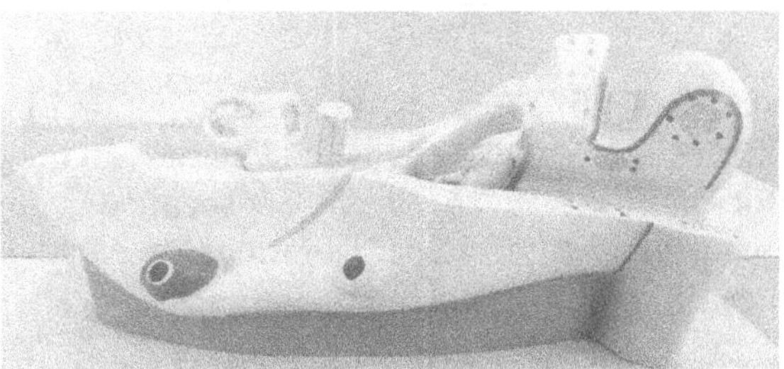

Observation: We learned the theory and anatomy of human ear using chart, specimen and models.

Result: The human ear has been studied with the help of chart, models, and specimens. The pictures are drawn and labelled.

Experiment No.: 36

Skin

Objective:	To study human skin with the help of chart, models, and specimens
Equipment/ Glassware Required:	Chart/model/specimen of human skin.

Principle

The skin is one of the largest organs in the body in surface area (20 square feet) and weight. The skin consists of three layers:

1. The epidermis: the outermost layer providing waterproof barrier and maintains the skin tone. The epidermis can be further subdivided into the following *strata* (beginning with the outermost layer): corneum, lucidum (only in palms of hands and bottoms of feet), granulosum, spinosum, and basale.

2. The dermis: It is present beneath the epidermis containing sweat glands, oil glands, connective tissue and hair follicles. The dermis is structurally divided into two areas: a superficial area adjacent to the epidermis, called the *papillary region*, and a deep thicker area known as the *reticular region*.

3. Hypodermis: it consists of fat and connective tissue.

The color of the skin is due to the presence of melanocytes which contains melanin pigment. These melanocytes are present in both dermis and epidermis. The thickness of the skin varies considerably over all parts of the body, and between men and women and the young and the old.

The skin has three main functions: protection, regulation and sensation. The primary function of is to act as a barrier and provides protection from: mechanical impacts and pressure, variations in temperature, micro-organisms, radiation and chemicals.

It regulates several aspects of physiology, including: body temperature via sweat and hair, and changes in peripheral circulation and fluid balance via sweat. It also acts as a reservoir for the synthesis of Vitamin D.

The skin contains an extensive network of nerve cells that detect and relay changes in the environment. Presence of separate receptors in skin help us to sense the heat, cold, touch, and pain.

Most common skin disorders include dermatitis, eczema, psoriasis, skin abscess, acne, herpes, melanoma, etc.

Procedure

Follow the below given steps:

- Collect chart, specimen and models of skin

- Observe different layers of the skin

- Identify subcutaneous layer of the skin

- Recognize hypodermis layer

- Differentiate sweat glands, sebaceous glands, adipose tissue and hair follicles.

- Draw the neat labelled diagram

- Record your observation

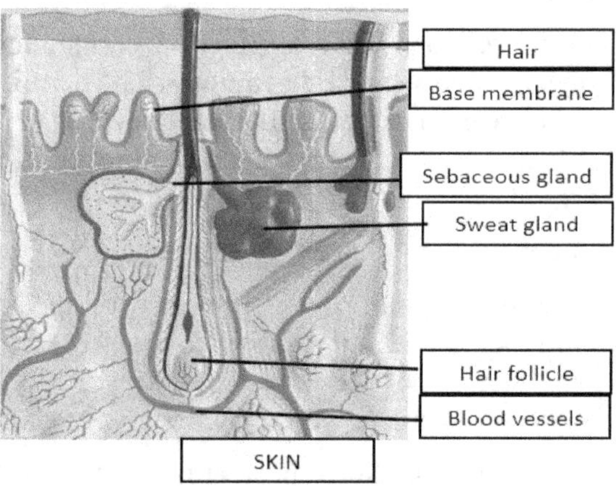

Observation: We learned the theory and anatomy of human skin using chart, specimen and models.

Result: Human skin has been studied with the help of chart, models, and specimens. The pictures are drawn and labelled.

Viva-voce

Q1. What do you mean by compound microscope?

ANS: The microscope which uses multiple lenses to magnify the image of a sample under observation.

Q2. What is the principle of compound microscope?

ANS: A virtual, inverted, and greatly magnified picture of the item is generated at the shortest distance of distinct vision from the eye held near to the eyepiece when the image of the object to be enlarged is positioned just outside the focus of its objective lens.

Q3. What should be the position of the condenser, when focusing at objective lens of 10x, 45x and 100x?

ANS: Move the condenser to its lowest position for 10x, midway for 45x and high for 100x.

Q4. In which condition do we use the concave and plane mirror of the microscope?

ANS: When a distant light source is present, the plane mirror is employed (For example, Natural day light). When the light source is close to the microscope, the concave mirror is utilised (For example, an electrical lamp).

Q5. Why do we use cedar wood oil in oil-immersion lens?

ANS: The specimen is covered in cedarwood oil to prevent refraction at the air-glass contact.

Q6. Name the parts of the fundamental elements of compound microscope.

ANS: The head, base, and arm are the three fundamental structural elements of a compound microscope.

Q7. What are the preventive measures taken for preventing the infection during venipuncture and skin pricking?

ANS: Elements of standard precautions relevant to venipuncture are hand hygiene, wearing non-sterile gloves, use of antiseptics – skin disinfection; cleaning and disinfection of materials used on more than one patient, including tourniquets, scissors and specimen carriers; disposal of used equipment, especially sharps.

Q8.   What are the sources and differences between venous blood and capillary blood?

ANS: In contrast to venous blood, capillary blood is closer to arterial blood. Capillary plasma has larger quantities of proteins, calcium, and chloride and lower amounts of potassium, sodium, and urea nitrogen when compared to venous plasma.

Q9.   What is the location and function of Simple Squamous epithelium?

ANS: Typically found lining blood veins and bodily cavities, this form of epithelium controls how chemicals enter the underlying tissue.

Q10.   What is the function of Simple Cuboidal epithelium?

ANS: They have a single layer of cuboidal cells with massive, centralised spherical nuclei. Their primary roles are secretion and absorption.

Q11.   What is the function of columnar epithelium?

ANS: This form of epithelium frequently features apical cilia or microvilli and is tailored for absorption.

Q12.   What is the function of Stratified squamous epithelium?

ANS: This kind of epithelium often performs defensive tasks, such as preventing bacteria from penetrating deeper tissues and/or preventing water loss.

Q13.   What is the function of Stratified cuboidal epithelium?

ANS: Stratified cuboidal epithelium, which may be seen in the sweat, mammary, and salivary glands, is often less prevalent. Protection, excretion, and secretion are their three main roles.

Q14.   What is the function of Stratified columnar epithelium?

ANS: This particular form of epithelium, which is both protective and mucus-secreting, is less frequent and is found in the mucous membrane (conjunctiva) lining of things like the eyelids.

Q15.   What the function is of stratified of transitional epithelium?

ANS: Transitional epithelium's stratified cells offer defence and let the vessels to enlarge to hold more body fluid.

Q16.   What are the features of skeletal muscles?

ANS: These muscle fibres run the whole length of the muscle. It perform a wide variety of actions because to the muscles' ability to move bones when their fibres contract (tighten).

Q17.   Name the regulatory proteins involved in contraction of muscles.

ANS: Actin and myosin.

Q18.   Which muscle is voluntary in nature?

ANS: Skeletal muscles

Q19.   Which type of muscle is not striated in appearance?

ANS: Smooth muscles

Q20.   Name the regulatory proteins in smooth muscle.

ANS: Tropomyosin (TM) and Caldesmon (CaD)

Q21.   What is the location and function of mesenchyme?

ANS: Numerous organs may contain mesenchymal tissues, which contribute to the strength and structure of the organs.

Q22.   What is the location and function of adipose tissue?

ANS: It's found under the skin (subcutaneous fat), between internal organs (visceral fat) and even in the inner cavities of bones (bone marrow adipose tissue).

Q23.   What is the location and function of dense regular connective tissue?

ANS: It is found in joint capsules, in the connective tissue that envelops muscles (muscle fascia), and it forms dermis of skin.

Q24.   What is the location and function of dense irregular connective tissue?

ANS: It is found in the skin's lowest layers (dermis) and the eyeball's protective white coating layer. Dense irregular fibrous connective tissue can be also found in joint capsules, the connective tissue that envelops muscles (muscle fascia), and the skin's dermis.

Q25.   What is the location and function of hyaline cartilage?

ANS: It is found at the ends of bones is sometimes referred to as articular cartilage. Hyaline cartilage is slippery and smooth which helps bones move smoothly past each other in joints.

Q26.   What is the location and function of elastic cartilage?

ANS: It is mostly located in the larynx, the pinna, and the tube that connects the centre of the ear to the throat. Elastic cartilage offers stability and has a medium degree of flexibility.

Q27.   What is the location and function of fibrocartilage?

ANS: It gives the tough substance for the intervertebral discs, the wrist, knee, and temporo-mandibular joints, as well as the articular cartilage of those joints and the junction between the clavicle and the sternum.

Q28.   How many bones are there in the adult skull? Name them.

ANS: In general, twenty-two bones make up the human skull: fourteen face skeleton bones and eight cranial bones. The occipital bone, two temporal bones, two parietal bones, the sphenoid, ethmoid, and frontal bones, as well as the two parietal bones, are all parts of the neurocranium.

Q29.   How many bones are there in vertebral column? Name them.

ANS: The vertebrae of the spine include the cervical spine (C1-C7), thoracic spine (T1-T12), lumbar spine (L1-L5), sacral spine (S1-S5), and the tailbone. Each vertebra is separated by a disc.

Q30.   How many bones are there in thorax? Name them.

ANS: The human thorax consists of the 12 thoracic vertebrae, 12 pairs of ribs, and the sternum.

Q31.   How many bones are there in the axial skeleton?

ANS: Axial skeleton is made up of the 80 bones

Q32.   Which is the weight-bearing bone of the leg?

ANS: The tibia is one of two bones that comprise the leg is weight-bearing bone.

Q33.   Which is the longest, heaviest & strongest bone in the body?

ANS: The femur

Q34.   Which is the triangular bone located anterior to the knee joint?

ANS: The patella

Q34.   Name the collar bone of the body.

ANS: The clavicular bone

Q35.   Name the parts of a typical vertebra.

ANS: A typical vertebra consists of a body and a vertebral arch

Q36.   Name the facial bones of the body.

ANS: Maxilla (2); Zygomatic (2); Mandible (1); Nasal (2); Platine (2); Inferior nasal concha (2); Lacrimal (2); Vomer (1)

Q37.   Name the cranial bones of the body.

ANS: Parietal (2); Temporal (2); Frontal (1); Occipital (1); Ethmoid (1); Sphenoid (1)

Q38.   Name the joints formed by humerus bones.

ANS: It articulates proximally with the glenoid via the glenohumeral (GH) joint and distally with the radius and ulna at the elbow joint.

Q39.   Name the joints formed by the femur with the pelvic bone.

ANS: The hip joint

Q40.   Name the joint formed by the clavicle with the scapula and sternum.

ANS: The Sternoclavicular Joint (SC joint)

Q36.   What is ABO Blood group?

ANS: A method for classifying distinct kinds of human blood according on whether or not the red blood cells' surfaces contain A and B antigens as markers.

Q37.   Which blood group person is a universal donor?

ANS: The blood group 'O'

Q38.   Which blood group person is the universal recipient?

ANS: The blood group 'AB'

Q39.   What is Rh system of blood group?

ANS: Red blood cells include the 5 primary Rh antigens C, c, D, E, and e. The Rh D is the most crucial of them. The positive (+) and the negative (-) after the letters A, B, AB, or O are determined by the presence or absence of the D antigen on the red cell, respectively.

Q40.   What is hemolytic disease of new born?

ANS: Hemolytic disease of the newborn (HDN) is a blood disorder in a fetus or newborn infant. In some infants, it can be fatal.

Q41.   Name the instrument used in determination of ESR.

ANS: Westergren apparatus

Q42.   What are the normal values of ESR?

ANS: Men under 50 years old: less than 15 mm/hr. Men over 50 years old: less than 20 mm/hr. Women under 50 years old: less than 20 mm/hr. Women over 50 years old: less than 30 mm/hr.

Q43.   What is the principle used in determination of Hb experiments?

ANS: Blood is mixed with N/10 HCl resulting in the conversion of Hb to acid hematin which is brown in color. The solution is diluted till it's color matches with the brown colored glass of the comparator box.

Q44.   What are the normal values of Hb in adult male and female?

ANS: For men, 13.2 to 16.6 grams per deciliter. For women, 11.6 to 15 grams per deciliter.

Q45.   How much blood is taken in Hb pipette?

ANS: 0.02 mL

Q46.   What do the yellow and red color readings signify in the Hb tube?

ANS: The hemoglobin tube is calibrated in g Hb% (2- 24 g%) in yellow color on one side and in percentage Hb (20- 140%) in red color on the other side.

Q47.   Name the dilution fluid used in RBC and WBC experiment?

ANS: Hayem's Fluid

Q48.   What is the difference between slow and fast speed pipette?

ANS: The capillary bore of RBC pipette is narrow, so it is slow speed pipette, whereas the capillary bore of WBC pipette is wider, hence it is a fast-speed pipette.

Q49.   What is the Neubauer improved chamber?

ANS: The Neubauer chamber is a thick crystal slide with the size of a glass slide (30 x 70 mm and 4 mm thickness) used for WBC and RBC count.

Q50.   What is the dimension of square in the counting grid of the Neubauer chamber?

ANS: Neubauer chamber's counting grid is 3 mm x 3 mm in size. The grid has 9 square subdivisions of width 1mm.

Q51.   What is the principle of determination of RBC and WBC experiment?

ANS: Principle for RBC experiment-The blood is diluted 200 times in red cell pipette and the cells are counted in the counting chamber. So, by knowing the dilution employed, their number in undiluted blood can be easily calculated.

Principle for WBC experiment- The sample of blood is diluted with a diluting fluid which destroys the red cells and stain the nuclei of the white blood cells. The cells are then counted in a counting chamber and their number in undiluted blood is determined.

Q52.   What is the dilution factor used in the RBC and WBC experiment?

ANS: For RBC is 200 and WBC is 20.

Q53.   How will you identify the RBC and WBC pipette?

ANS: The RBC pipette is identified by the red bead in the bulb, mouth piece is red in color and just beyond the bulb, the number 101 is etched on the RBC pipette. For the WBC pipette by the white bead in the bulb, mouth piece is white in color and the just beyond the bulb, the number 11 is etched on the WBC pipette

Q54. Define blood pressure?

ANS: The force exerted by blood on blood vessels while flowing through it.

Q55. Name the apparatus used is determination of blood pressure.

ANS: Sphygmomanometer

Q56. Define systolic and diastolic blood pressure.

ANS: Systolic blood pressure, measures the pressure in arteries by blood during systolic phase of heart. Diastolic blood pressure, measures the pressure in arteries by blood during diastole of the heart.

Q57. What is the normal value of blood pressure?

ANS: 120/80 in adults

Q58. How will you measure body temperature?

ANS: Using thermometer

Q59. What is the normal respiratory rate of an adult?

ANS: 12 to 16 breaths per minute.

Q60. How will you measure the pulse rate? What is the normal value?

ANS: Use first and second fingertips, press firmly but gently on the arteries until feel a pulse. Begin counting the pulse for 60 seconds. 60-100 beats per minute.

Q61. Define tidal volume and vital capacity of lungs?

ANS: Tidal volume is the amount of air that moves in or out of the lungs with each respiratory cycle. Vital capacity is the volume of air that is expelled from the lung during a maximal forced expiration effort starting after a maximal forced inspiration (4.5L).

Q62. What is minute ventilation?

ANS: Minute ventilation is the volume of gas inhaled (inhaled minute volume) or exhaled (exhaled minute volume) from a person's lungs per minute.

Q63. What is the formula of BMI?

ANS: Weight in kilograms divided by height in meters squared

Q64. What is the normal value of BMI in adults?

ANS: An ideal BMI is in the 18.5 to 24.9 range.

Q65. What is the location of the heart?

ANS: It is located in the front of chest, slightly behind and to the left of sternum

Q66.   Name the chambers and valves in the heart.

ANS: Chambers: Right atrium, Right ventricle, Left atrium, Left ventricle
        Valves: Tricuspid valve, Pulmonary valve, Mitral valve, Aortic valve.

Q67.   Why is the left ventricle thicker than the right ventricle?

ANS: The left ventricle pump blood for the systemic circulation. Because of this
        it has the largest, most muscular walls of any of the chambers.

Q68.   What is cardiac output?

ANS: Cardiac output is the product of heart rate (HR) and stroke volume (SV)
        and is measured in liters per minute.

Q69.   Name the parts of the respiratory system?

ANS: The respiratory system includes the nose, mouth, throat, voice box,
        windpipe, lungs, and diaphragm.

Q70.   How many lobes are there in the right and left lungs?

ANS: The right lung consists of three and left lung consists of two lobes.

Q71.   What is alveoli?

ANS: These are tiny air sacs at the end of the bronchioles

Q72.   Name the parts of the digestive system.

ANS: Mouth, esophagus, stomach, small intestine, large intestine, liver,
        pancreas, gallbladder and anus.

Q73.   What is the role of the stomach?

ANS: It takes in food from the esophagus, mixes it, breaks it down, and then
        passes it on to the small intestine in small portions.

Q74.   Name the parts of accessory digestive organs.

ANS: The accessory organs are the teeth, tongue, and glandular organs such as
        salivary glands, liver, gallbladder, and pancreas.

Q75.   What is the role of bile in digestion of food?

ANS: It breaks down fats into fatty acids, which can be easy to absorb by the
        digestive tract.

Q76.   Name the enzymes released from pancreas.

ANS: Pancreatic Amylase, Pancreatic Protease(trypsin), Pancreatic Lipase

Q77.   Name the brush border enzymes.

ANS: Maltase-glucoamylase and sucrase-isomaltase are closely related enzymes
        embedded in the brush border membrane

Q78.   Name the parts of brain.

ANS: The brain can be divided into three basic units: the forebrain, the midbrain, and the hindbrain.

Q79.   What are the functions of cerebrum, pons, medulla oblongata?

ANS: Cerebrum initiates and coordinates movement and regulates temperature, enable speech, judgment, thinking and reasoning, problem-solving, emotions, learning, vision, hearing, touch and other senses.

The pons is the origin for four of the 12 cranial nerves, involved in tear production, chewing, blinking, focusing vision, balance, hearing and facial expression.

Functions of the medulla regulate many bodily activities, including heart rhythm, breathing, blood flow, and oxygen and carbon dioxide levels. It produces reflexive activities such as sneezing, vomiting, coughing and swallowing.

Q80.   Name the endocrine glands of the body.

ANS: Pituitary, thyroid, parathyroid, thymus, and adrenal glands

Q81.   Why pituitary gland called as master gland of the body?

ANS: Because it controls the functions of many of the other endocrine glands

Q82.   What are the functions of growth hormone?

ANS: Influencing growth of height, build bones and muscles

Q83.   What are the functions of thyroid hormones?

ANS: The thyroid gland produces hormones that regulate the body's metabolic rate controlling heart, muscle and digestive function, brain development and bone maintenance.

Q84.   What is the function of aldosterone?

ANS: It helps control the balance of water and salts in the kidney by keeping sodium in and releasing potassium from the body.

Q85.   What are gluco corticosteroids?

ANS: These are the steroid hormones widely used for the treatment of inflammation, autoimmune diseases, and cancer.

Q86.   What is the role of insulin and glucagon in the body?

ANS: These are involved in regulating blood glucose levels.

Q87. Name the parts of male reproductive system.

ANS: The male reproductive system contains the external genitals the penis, testes and the scrotum; and internal parts, including the prostate gland, vas deferens and urethra.

Q88. Name the parts of the female reproductive system.

ANS: It include the uterus, ovaries, fallopian tubes, cervix, and vagina.

Q89. Name the hormone released from testis.

ANS: Testosterone

Q90. Name the hormone released from the ovary.

ANS: Estrogen and progesterone

Q91. What is the role of testosterone in the body?

ANS: Testosterone is a male sex hormone regulate sex drive (libido), bone mass, fat distribution, muscle mass and strength, and the production of red blood cells and sperm

Q92. What is the role of estrogen and progesterone in the body?

ANS: One primary action of these hormones is to regulate the development and function of the uterus.

Q93. Name the parts of the eye.

ANS: Sclera, Cornea, Iris, Pupil, Lens, Retina, and Optic nerves.

Q94. What is the role of iris and lens in the eye?

ANS: The iris controls the amount of light the pupil gets and lens focus light correctly on the retina.

Q95. Where is the image formed in the eyes?

ANS: Retina

Q96. Name the parts of the ear.

ANS: Outer Ear, Middle Ear, Inner Ear and auditory nerve.

Q97. Name the part of the inner ear responsible for maintaining balance of the body.

ANS: Vestibular system

Q98. Name the part of the inner ear responsible for maintaining hearing.

ANS: Cochlea

Q99. Name the various layers of epidermis.

ANS: The layers of the epidermis include the stratum basale, stratum spinosum, stratum granulosum, stratum lucidum, and stratum corneum.

Q100.   What are the various functions of skin?

ANS: Provides a protective barrier against mechanical, thermal and physical injury and hazardous substances.

Q101.   What is the role of keratin and melanin in the skin?

ANS: Keratin is a protein that helps form hair, nails and your skin's outer layer (epidermis). Melanin provides the pigment in skin, hair and eyes.

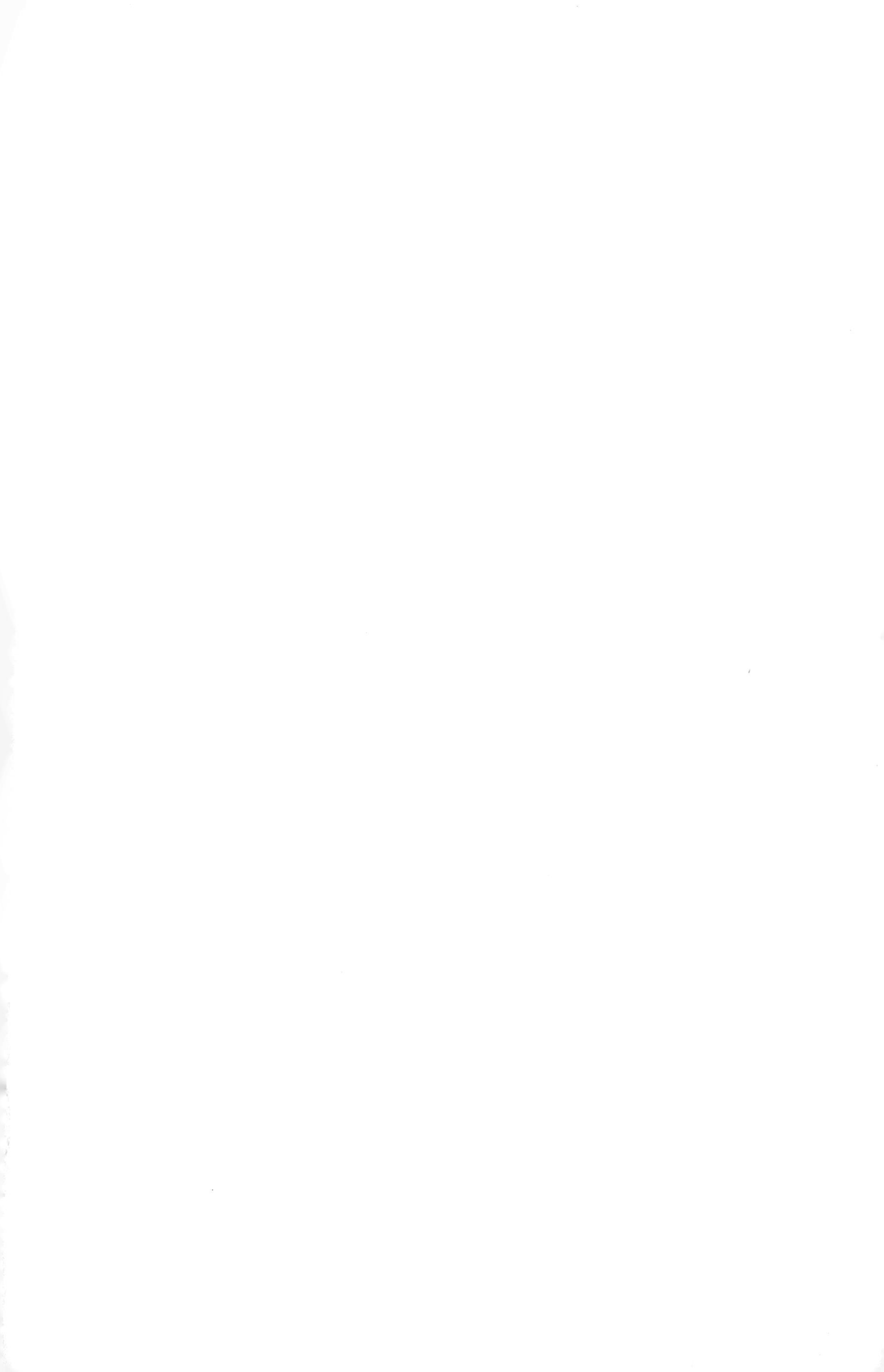